Laboratory Manual

to accompany

Therapeutic Modalities for Sports Medicine and Athletic Training

Fifth Edition

William E. Prentice, Ph.D., P.T., A.T.C.
The University of North Carolina at Chapel Hill

Prepared by

William S. Quillen, Ph.D., P.T., S.C.S.
Indiana University School of Medicine
Indianapolis, Indiana

Frank B. Underwood, Ph.D., M.P.T., E.C.S.
The University of Evansville
Evansville, Indiana

Boston   Burr Ridge, IL   Dubuque, IA   Madison, WI   New York   San Francisco   St. Louis
Bangkok   Bogotá   Caracas   Kuala Lumpur   Lisbon   London   Madrid   Mexico City
Milan   Montreal   New Delhi   Santiago   Seoul   Singapore   Sydney   Taipei   Toronto

McGraw-Hill Higher Education ⚛

A Division of The McGraw-Hill Companies

Laboratory Manual to accompany
Therapeutic Modalities for Sports Medicine and Athletic Training, Fifth Edition
William E. Prentice

Published by McGraw-Hill Higher Education, an imprint of The McGraw-Hill Companies, Inc., 1221 Avenue of the Americas, New York, NY 10020. Copyright © The McGraw-Hill Companies, Inc., 2003, 1999, 1995. All rights reserved.

This book is printed on acid-free paper.

1 2 3 4 5 6 7 8 9 0 QPD QPD 0 3 2

ISBN 0-07-246212-4

www.mhhe.com

Preface

We continue to be gratified by the response to our *Laboratory Manual to accompany THERAPEUTIC MODALITIES FOR SPORTS MEDICINE AND ATHLETIC TRAINING.* With the subsequent publication of the 5th edition of Prentice's text, we have once again set about to incorporate suggestions received from reviewers and users in the field to enhance the manual's utility as a first practical workbook to guide the user to competency in the basic application of physical agent modalities. With the incorporation of additional case studies and discussion questions at the end of each chapter, the student is encouraged to link the ***how*** of application learned through this manual with the necessary ***why*** found in the textbook. Knowledge in the employment and consistency in the application of physical agent interventions is the key to professional care and a successful and satisfactory outcome.

WSQ
FBU

Contents

How to Use This Laboratory Manual

This laboratory manual is designed to be used with the textbook, *Therapeutic Modalities for Sports Medicine and Athletic Training, 5th edition*. Theory, biophysical principles and range of potential sports medicine applications for the various physical agent modalities will be found in that text. This manual is intended to provide the student or interested reader with a systematic and sequential method of completing a basic physical agent modality application. The initial performance of a therapeutic procedure should proceed in a logical step-wise fashion. This manual is structured to allow both the instructor or supervisor and the student the ability to assess competency in a partial or complete fashion culminating in the independent ability to safely and effectively provide a physical agent modality intervention.

Each physical agent modality application has a separate sequential checklist. Similarities will be noted in certain aspects of treatment application and completion. Space is provided for up to three separate instructors/supervisors to "sign off" (initial and date) the successful completion and demonstration of each element of the complete application. A **Master Competency Check List** is provided at the beginning of the manual to document the successful completion of the individual physical agent modality checklist and when the student is deemed competent to independently provide that intervention. This system documents the acquisition of fundamental skills necessary for effective physical agent modality application and ensures accountability by the student and instructor/supervisor to patients and other concerned parties.

Competency in the skillful application of physical agent modalities is gained through diligent and frequent practice. Use of this manual in the manner described will guide the user in productive practice and successful acquisition of essential skills. Students are encouraged to practice each of the procedures on themselves first; thereby gaining an appreciation of the sensations associated with that particular physical agent. Further practice with a variety of lab partners will result in the development of the desired competence and confidence with any manufacturer's equipment.

Master Competency Checklist

PHYSICAL AGENT MODALITY	Examiner		
	1	2	3
Positioning			
Electrical Stimulation			
Analgesia			
Muscle Reeducation			
Muscle Strengthening			
Iontophoresis			
Biofeedback			
Shortwave Diathermy			
Infrared Physical Agents			
Thermotherapy			
Hydrocollator Pack			
Paraffin Bath			
Infrared Lamp			
Cryotherapy			
Ice Massage			
Ice Pack			
Gel Cold Pack			
Vapocoolant Spray			
Hydrotherapy			
Warm Whirlpool			
Cold Whirlpool			
Contrast Bath			

Checklist continues

PHYSICAL AGENT MODALITY	Examiner		
	1	2	3
Fluidotherapy®			
Ultraviolet			
Low-Power Laser			
Ultrasound			
Direct Contact			
Bladder Coupling			
Underwater Coupling			
Phonophoresis			
Mechanical Traction			
Cervical			
Lumbar			
Intermittent Compression			
Massage			

Chapter 1: GUIDELINES FOR USING PHYSICAL AGENT MODALITIES

- *ROLE OF PHYSICAL AGENT MODALITIES*

The therapist employs physical agent modalities to create an optimum environment for tissue healing while minimizing the symptoms associated with neuromusculoskeletal trauma.

- *SYMPTOMS OF NEUROMUSCULOSKELETAL TRAUMA*

Pain
Muscle Spasm
Warmth/Erythema
Soft Tissue Edema - Articular Effusion
Muscle and/or Joint Dysfunction

- *PHASES OF INJURY – HEALING CONTINUUM* (See Table 1-1)

Acute Injury Phase
Inflammatory Response Phase
Fibroblastic Repair Phase
Maturation - Remodeling Phase

- *CLINICAL DECISION MAKING* (See Table 1-2)

What tissues are Injured/Affected?
    Contractile
    Non-contractile

What Symptoms are Present?

What Phase of Injury – Healing Continuum?

What are Physical Agent Modality's Biophysical Effects?
    Direct Effects
    Indirect Effects
    Depth of Penetration
    Tissue Affinity

What are Physical Agent Modality's Indications?

What are Physical Agent Modality's Contraindications?

Resources Available in Your Facility?
    Cyrotherapy
      Cold Packs
      Ice Massage
      Gel Cold Packs
      Vapocoolant Spray
    Thermotherapy
      Paraffin
      Hydrocollator Pack
      Infrared Lamp
    Electrical Stimulating Currents
      Low-Voltage Galvanic
      Iontophoresis
      Pulsatile Monophasic
      Medium Frequency Polyphasic
      Interferential
    Intermittent Compression
    Diathermy
      Microwave
      Shortwave
    Ultraviolet
    Low-Power Laser
    Ultrasound
      Pulsed
      Continuous
      1 or 3 MHz
      Phonophoresis

What are the Parameters of Physical Agents Modality's Application?
    Dosage
    Duration
    Frequency

• *CHOICE OF PHYSICAL AGENT MODALITY*

Table 1-1
Critical Decision Making on the Use of Various Therapeutic Modalities in Treatment of Acute Injury

Phase	Approximate Time Frame	Clinical Picture	Possible Modalities Used	Rationale for Use
Initial acute	Injury—day 3	Swelling, pain to touch, pain on motion	CRYO	↓ Swelling, ↓Pain
			ESC	↓ Pain
			IC	↓ Swelling
				↓ Pain
			ULTRA	Nonthermal effects to ↑ healing
Inflammatory Response	Day 2—day 6	Swelling subsides, warm to touch, discoloration, pain to touch, pain on motion	CRYO	↓ Swelling, ↓Pain
			ESC	↓ Pain
			IC	↓ Swelling
				↓ Pain
			ULTRA	Nonthermal effects to ↑ healing
			Range of motion	
Fibroblastic-Repair	Day 4—day 10	Pain to touch, pain on motion, swollen	THERMO	Mildly ↑ circulation
			ESC	↓ Pain—muscle pumping
				↓ Pain
			IC	Facilitate lymphatic flow
			ULTRA	Nonthermal effects to ↑ healing
			Range of motion	
			Strengthening	
Maturation Remodeling	Day 7—recovery	Swollen, no more pain to touch, decreasing pain on motion	ULTRA	Deep heating to ↑ circulation
			ESC	↑ Range of motion, ↑ strength
				↓ Pain
			SWD	↓ Pain
			MWD	Deep heating to ↑ circulation
			Range of motion	Deep heating to ↑ circulation
			Strengthening	
			Functional activities	

CYRO, Cryotherapy; ESC, electrical stimulating currents; IC, intermittent compression; MWD, microwave diathermy; SWD, shortwave diathermy; THERMO, thermotherapy; ULTRA, ultrasound; ↓ decrease; ↑ increase

3

TABLE 1-2
Indications and Contraindications for Therapeutic Modalities

Therapeutic Modality	Physiological Responses (Indications for Use)	Contraindications and Precautions
Electrical stimulating currents—Pulsatile Monophasic	Pain modulation Muscle reeducation Muscle pumping contractions Retard atrophy Muscle strengthening Increase range of motion Fracture healing Acute injury	Pacemakers Thrombophlebitis Superficial skin lesions
Electrical stimulating currents—Low-voltage	Wound healing Fracture healing Iontophoresis	Malignancy Skin hypersensitivities Allergies to certain drugs
Electrical stimulating currents—Interferential	Pain modulation Muscle reeducation Muscle pumping contractions Fracture healing Increase range of motion	Same as high-voltage
Electrical stimulating currents—Medium Frequency	Muscle strengthening	Pacemakers

4

Therapeutic Modality	Physiological Responses (Indications for Use)	Contraindications and Precautions
Shortwave diathermy and Microwave diathermy	Increase deep circulation Increase metabolical activity Reduce muscle guarding/spasm Reduce inflammation Facilitate wound healing Analgesia Increase tissue temperatures over a large area	Metal implants Pacemakers Malignancy Wet dressings Anesthetized areas Pregnancy Acute injury and inflammation Eyes Areas of reduced blood flow Anesthetized area
Cryotherapy—cold packs, Ice massage	Acute injury Vasoconstriction—decreased blood flow Analgesia Reduce inflammation Increase metabolical activity Facilitate tissue healing	Acute and postacute trauma Poor circulation Circulatory impairments Malignancy
Thermotherapy—hot whirlpool, paraffin, hydrocollator, infrared lamps	Vasodilation—increased blood flow Analgesia Reduce muscle guarding/spasm Reduce inflammation Increase metabolical activity Facilitate tissue healing	Allergy to cold Circulatory impairments Wound healing Hypertension
Ultraviolet	Acne Aseptic wounds Folliculitis Pityriasis rosea Tinea Septic wounds Sinusitis Increase calcium metabolism	Psoriasis Eczema Herpes Diabetes Pellagra Lupus erythematosus Hyperthyroidism Renal and hepatic insufficiency Generalized dermatitis Advanced arteriosclerosis

Therapeutic Modality	Physiological Responses (Indications for Use)	Contraindications and Precautions
Ultrasound	Increase connective tissue extensibility Deep heat Increased circulation Treatment of most soft tissue injuries Reduce inflammation Reduce muscle spasm	Infection Acute and postacute injury Epiphyseal areas Pregnancy Thrombophlebitis Impaired sensation Eyes
Intermittent compression	Decrease acute bleeding Decrease edema	Circulatory impairment

Chapter 2: PATIENT POSITIONING

DESCRIPTION:

The positioning of a patient prior to the application of a physical agent modality is one of the most important aspects contributing to a successful treatment. Placing the patient in an aligned and supported position insures muscular relaxation and facilitates venous flow of blood. Proper positioning allows the use of optimal body mechanics by the sports therapist in the application of the selected treatment.

THERAPEUTIC EFFECTS:
- Muscular Relaxation
- Facilitated Venous Blood Flow

When performing the tasks on the Patient Positioning checklist refer to the following illustrations:

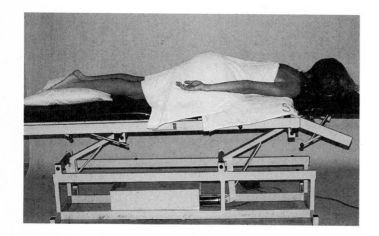
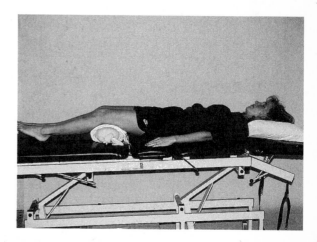
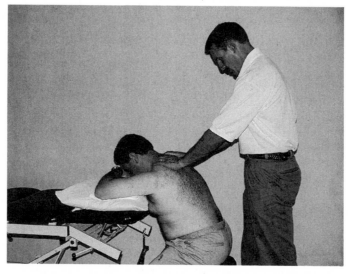

PATIENT POSITIONING

PROCEDURE	Evaluation #		
	1	2	3
1. Check Supplies			
a. Pillows			
b. Towels			
c. Sheets			
2. Question Patient			
a. Verify Identity			
b. Verify Treatment Area			
3. Position Patient			
a. Prone on Table (Figure 2-1)			
1. Place Pillow Under Abdomen - Lumbar Spine Should be Flat			
2. Place Pillow Under Ankles			
3. Insure Proper Body Alignment			
4. Drape Patient to Maintain Modesty			
b. Supine (Figure 2-2)			
1. Place Pillow Under Head and Knees			
2. Insure Proper Body Alignment			
3. Drape Patient to Maintain Modesty			
c. Sitting (Figure 2-3)			
1. Seat Patient on Chair or Stool Leaning Forward			
2. Support Head and Shoulders with Pillows			
3. Rest Forearms and Hands on Table			
4. Insure Proper Body Alignment			
5. Drape Patient to Maintain Modesty			

Checklist continues

PROCEDURE	Evaluation #		
	1	2	3
4. Administer the Treatment			
5. Complete the Treatment			
6. Return Equipment to Storage After Cleaning			

Chapter 3: ELECTRICAL STIMULATION
ANALGESIA

DESCRIPTION:

Electroanalgesia is arguably the most common use of therapeutic electricity. The use of therapeutic electricity for analgesia is often referred to as Transcutaneous Electrical Nerve Stimulation or TENS; however, all forms of therapeutic electricity that do not use implanted or needle electrodes are "transcutaneous", and many forms stimulate nerves. Therefore, the term "TENS" should be discouraged. Although there are hundreds of different types of electrical stimulators available for use, there are essentially three levels in the body that may be affected.

The first level is the spinal gate. This level is activated by increasing the input to the spinal cord from large diameter afferent neurons. The second level is referred to as the central bias mechanism, where intense small fiber afferent input activates a negative feedback loop through connections in the mid-brain. Finally, some forms of electrical stimulation appear to stimulate the production of endogenous opiates, the endorphins.

Although stimulators have many different waveforms and modulations, there is no evidence that an "optimal" waveform exists. It is impossible to predict for an individual patient what type of current, what electrode configuration, what amplitude of stimulation, etc., will provide relief of pain. Therefore, electroanalgesia is somewhat of a trial and error phenomenon. This does not mean the approach should be haphazard; a systematic approach, based on clinical experience is best.

Generally, there are three types of stimulation for electroanalgesia; conventional, low frequency, and hyperstimulation. Conventional generally has a pulse rate of 10 to 100 pulses per second (pps), and is applied at an amplitude between sensory and motor thresholds. Low frequency stimulation has a pulse rate of one to five pps, and an amplitude between motor and pain thresholds. Hyperstimulation generally uses a monophasic pulsatile current at a frequency of 1 to 128 pps, and an amplitude to pain tolerance. Hyperstimulation is often referred to as "point stimulation."

PHYSIOLOGICAL EFFECTS:

• Depolarization of peripheral nerves

THERAPEUTIC EFFECTS:

• Inhibition of pain perception

INDICATIONS:

The obvious indication for electroanalgesia is pain. However, the cause of the pain should be identified prior to the use of electrical stimulation, and it must be remembered that the modulation of pain is not treating the cause of the pain.

CONTRAINDICATIONS:

- Pregnancy
- Implanted electrical pacing devices (e.g., cardiac pacemaker, bladder stimulator, etc.)
- Cardiac arrhythmia
- Over the carotid sinus area
- Hypersensitivity (i.e., the patient who has a strong aversion to electricity, or the patient with certain types of catheters or shunts).

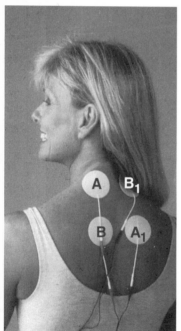

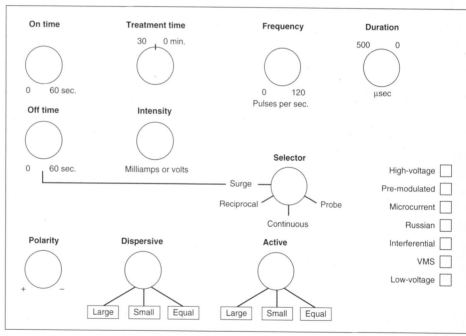

ELECTRICAL STIMULATION: ANALGESIA

PROCEDURE	Evaluation #		
	1	2	3
1. Check supplies			
a. Obtain towels or sheets for draping, conductant.			
b. Check stimulator, electrodes, and cables for charged battery, broken or frayed insulation, etc.			
c. Insure the amplitude controls are at zero.			
2. Question patient			
a. Verify identity of patient (if not already verified).			
b. Verify the absence of contraindications.			
c. Ask about previous treatments for current condition, and check treatment notes.			
3. Position patient			
a. Place patient in a well-supported, comfortable position.			
b. Expose body part to be treated.			
c. Drape patient to preserve patient's modesty, protect clothing, but allow access to body part.			
4. Inspect body part to be treated			
a. Check light touch perception.			
b. Assess function of body part (e.g., ROM, irritability).			

Checklist continues

PROCEDURE	Evaluation #		
	1	2	3
5a. Apply conventional electrical stimulation			
a. Place conductant on electrodes as indicated, secure electrodes to patient.			
b. Remind the patient to inform you when they feel something. Do not tell the patient what they will feel; e.g., do not say, "tell me when you feel a buzz or tingle."			
c. Adjust the pulse rate, pulse width, and mode of stimulation to desired settings if possible.			
d. Turn on the stimulator, and increase the amplitude slowly. Monitor the patient's response, not the stimulator.			
e. After the patient reports the onset of the stimulus, adjust the amplitude to a comfortable level, but make sure it is below motor threshold. If it is impossible to achieve supra-sensory threshold stimulation without a motor response, turn the stimulator off and move the electrodes to another location.			
f. Set a timer for the appropriate treatment time and give the patient a signaling device. Make sure the patient understands how to use the signaling device.			
g. Recheck the patient after about five minutes. If the sensation has diminished, adjust the amplitude appropriately.			

Checklist continues

PROCEDURE	Evaluation #		
	1	2	3
5b. Apply low frequency electrical stimulation			
a. Place conductant on electrodes as indicated, secure electrodes to patient.			
b. Remind the patient to inform you when they feel something. Do not tell the patient what they will feel; e.g., do not say, "tell me when you feel a buzz or tingle."			
c. Adjust the pulse rate, pulse width, and mode of stimulation to desired settings if possible.			
d. Turn on the stimulator, and increase the amplitude slowly. Monitor the patient's response, not the stimulator.			
e. After the patient reports the onset of the stimulus, adjust the amplitude to a comfortable level above motor threshold. The contraction should be just a twitch, not a strong contraction.			
f. Set a timer for the appropriate treatment time and give the patient a signaling device. Make sure the patient understands how to use the signaling device.			
g. Recheck the patient after about five minutes. If the sensation has diminished, adjust the amplitude appropriately.			

Checklist continues

PROCEDURE	Evaluation #		
	1	2	3
5c. Apply hyperstimulation electrical stimulation			
a. Place conductant on "inactive" electrode, have patient hold electrode in palm. Apply conductant to points to be stimulated.			
b. If using electrical resistance to locate stimulation points, set sensitivity of ohmmeter; set pulse rate, polarity, and length of stimulation to desired settings.			
c. Move the "active" electrode slowly in the area of the point to be stimulated until the area of minimal resistance is found; the pressure applied to the electrode must be constant.			
d. Tell the patient to report when the amplitude of stimulation is as high as they can tolerate. Activate the stimulation current, and increase the amplitude slowly. Monitor the patient's response, not the stimulator.			
e. After the patient reports that the stimulus is as much as they can tolerate, maintain constant pressure on the electrode. Stimulate the point two or three times, for 15 to 30 seconds each time.			

Checklist continues

PROCEDURE	Evaluation #		
	1	2	3
f. Repeat the process for each point to be stimulated.			
6. Complete treatment			
a. When the treatment time is over, turn the intensity control to zero, and move the generator away from the patient; remove conductant with a towel.			
b. Remove material used for draping, assist the patient in dressing as needed.			
c. Have the patient perform appropriate therapeutic exercise as indicated.			
d. Clean the treatment area and equipment according to normal protocol.			
7. Assess treatment efficacy			
a. Ask the patient how the treated area feels.			
b. Visually inspect the treated area for any adverse reactions.			
c. Perform functional tests as indicated.			

Case Study #1: ELECTRICAL STIMULATION: ANALGESIA

Background: A 52-year-old woman is 9 months post hemilaminectomy and discectomy without fusion at L5-S1 due to a herniated disc with compromise of the S1 nerve root. The surgery resulted in relief of the peripheral pain, weakness, and sensory loss, but persistent pain in the lumbosacral spine and buttock prevents the patient from engaging in rehabilitation exercises effectively.

Impression: Status-post spinal surgery with persistent post-operative pain; no neural deficit.

Treatment Plan: The patient was already being treated with a hot pack prior to exercise; conventional TENS was added to the treatment regimen. Electrodes were placed at the L3-4 interspace and over the greater trochanter. A pulsatile biphasic waveform was selected, with a rate of 60 pps, amplitude between the sensory and motor thresholds, and a duty cycle of 1:0 (uninterrupted). The stimulation was delivered for the 10-minute heat application, and remained in place during the therapeutic exercise, as well as for 30 minutes following the exercise.

Response: The patient experienced a 60% reduction in the symptoms during the treatment; this enabled the patient to perform the exercise through a greater range and with a greater effect. The effect of the TENS began to diminish after 8 weeks, but the pain had diminished to manageable levels such that the patient was able to continue the rehabilitation program without the TENS.

Case Study #2: ELECTRICAL STIMULATION: ANALGESIA

Background: A 47-year-old man sustained a closed crush injury of the right foot in a construction accident 12 weeks ago. Radiographs revealed no bony injury, and the physical examination indicated that the neurovascular structures were intact. A pneumatic immobilization device was applied to the right leg in the emergency department, the patient was supplied with axillary crutches, and he was instructed to avoid weight bearing on the right foot until he was cleared by his family physician. The immobilization device was removed six weeks ago, and the patient was instructed to begin progressive weight bearing and to exercise the foot on his own. He has now been referred to you because of a progressive increase in burning pain in the foot and leg, with swelling and extreme sensitivity to touch. The patient refuses to bear weight on the foot, and is not wearing a sock or shoe on the right foot.

Impression: Complex Regional Pain Syndrome type I (aka Reflex Sympathetic Dystrophy).

Treatment Plan: A pulsatile biphasic current was delivered to the right leg, with electrodes over the anterior and posterior compartments. The frequency was 2 pps, and the amplitude was above the patient's pain threshold, but below pain tolerance; a strong muscular twitch response was elicited. The current was delivered without interruption (duty cycle of 1:0) for 60 seconds. When the current was turned off, the patient's foot was brushed lightly with the therapist's hands. The process was repeated a total of 10 times in the initial treatment session, and the patient was instructed to attempt the brushing process at home.

Response: After the initial 60 seconds of current at the first treatment session, the patient was able to tolerate five seconds of light touch. After the 10th period of stimulation, the patient was able to tolerate 45 seconds of moderate touch. Treatment was repeated three days per week for two weeks, at which time the patient was able to tolerate a sock and shoe, was partial weight-bearing, and continued the desensitization process on a home program.

Discussion Questions for Case Studies

- What tissues were injured/affected?

- What symptoms were present?

- What phase of the injury – healing continuum did the patient present for care in?

- What are the physical agent modality's biophysical effects? (direct/indirect/depth/tissue affinity)

- What are the physical agent modality's indications/contraindications?

- What are the parameters of the physical agent modality's application/dosage/duration/frequency in this case study?

The rehabilitation professional employs physical agent modalities to create an optimum environment for tissue healing while minimizing the symptoms associated with the trauma or condition.

What other physical agent modalities could be utilized to treat this injury or condition? Why? How?

Further Discussion Questions

- What factors led to the selection of conventional TENS?

- What would be the advantages and disadvantages of low-TENS for this patient?

- What is the theoretical mechanism of action of conventional TENS?

- Why did the effect of the TENS diminish over time?

- Would you characterize the patient's pain as chronic or acute? Why? Are there different optimum forms of electrical stimulation for pain relief dependent upon the nature of the pain?

- What is Complex Regional Pain Syndrome (CRPS) type I?

- What is the difference between CRPS type I and CRPS type II?

- Why was low frequency TENS selected for this patient? Would other forms of TENS (e.g., conventional, hyperstimulation) have been effective? Why or why not?

- Is it likely that CRPS could have been prevented in this patient? How?

ELECTRICAL STIMULATION: MUSCLE REEDUCATION

DESCRIPTION:

Electrical stimulation may be used to HELP a patient in regaining the ability to voluntarily control a normally innervated muscle. Sometimes following surgery, a patient temporarily loses the ability to produce a muscle contraction. Probably the most common loss is of the quadriceps femoris following knee surgery. In addition, if a patient has undergone a tendon transfer, they may have difficulty recruiting the muscle to perform the new joint action.

The mechanism by which electrical stimulation aids in the recovery of volitional control of skeletal muscle is not clear. However, the reason volitional control is lost following surgery is not clear either. The probable method of action is via stimulation of joint, muscle, and skin proprioceptors when the muscle produces joint motion.

PHYSIOLOGICAL EFFECTS:

- Depolarization of peripheral nerves

THERAPEUTIC EFFECTS:

- Recovery of volitional control of skeletal muscle

INDICATIONS:

The primary indication is loss of volitional control of a skeletal muscle following surgery or a tendon transfer.

CONTRAINDICATIONS:

- Pregnancy
- Implanted electrical pacing devices (e.g., cardiac pacemaker, bladder stimulator, etc.)
- Cardiac arrhythmia
- Over the carotid sinus area
- Hypersensitivity (i.e., the patient who has a strong aversion to electricity, or the patient with certain types of catheters or shunts).

ELECTRICAL STIMULATION: MUSCLE REEDUCATION

PROCEDURE	Evaluation #		
	1	2	3
1. Check supplies			
a. Obtain towels or sheets for draping, conductant.			
b. Check stimulator, electrodes, and cables for charged battery, broken or frayed insulation, etc.			
c. Verify that the intensity control is at zero.			
2. Question patient			
a. Verify identity of patient (if not already verified).			
b. Verify the absence of contraindications.			
c. Ask about previous exposure to electrotherapy, check treatment notes.			
3. Position patient			
a. Place patient in a well-supported, comfortable position.			
b. Expose body part to be treated.			
c. Drape patient to preserve patient's modesty, protect clothing, but allow access to body part.			
4. Inspect body part to be treated			
a. Check light touch perception.			
b. Assess function of body part (e.g., ROM, irritability).			

Checklist continues

PROCEDURE	Evaluation #		
	1	2	3
5. Apply electrical stimulation for re-education			
a. Place conductant on electrodes as needed, secure electrodes to patient. Electrode location will vary depending on desired effect. Usually, the ideal location for the active electrode is over the motor point of the target muscle, or the peripheral nerve trunk that supplies the target muscle.			
b. Remind the patient to inform you when they feel something. Do not tell the patient what they will feel; e.g., do not say "tell me when you feel a buzz or tingle."			
c. Adjust the pulse rate, pulse width, and mode of stimulation to desired settings if possible.			
d. Turn on the stimulator, and increase the amplitude slowly. Monitor the patient's response, not the stimulator.			
e. After the patient reports the onset of the stimulus, adjust the amplitude to a comfortable level above motor threshold. Encourage the patient to try to volitionally contract the muscle before the stimulator does, and increase the force during the stimulation.			

Checklist continues

PROCEDURE	Evaluation #		
	1	2	3
f. Continue to monitor the patient during the duration of the treatment.			
6. Complete treatment			
a. When the treatment time is over or the patient is able to control the muscle contraction, turn the intensity to zero, and move the generator away from the patient; remove conductant with a towel.			
b. Remove material used for draping, assist the patient in dressing as needed.			
c. Have the patient perform appropriate therapeutic exercise as indicated.			
d. Clean the treatment area and equipment according to normal protocol.			
7. Assess treatment efficacy			
a. Ask the patient how the treated area feels.			
b. Visually inspect the treated area for any adverse reactions.			
c. Perform functional tests as indicated.			

Case Study #1: ELECTRICAL STIMULATION: MUSCLE REEDUCATION

Background: A 16 year-old male underwent arthroscopic partial medial meniscectomy on the right knee yesterday. He is to begin ambulation with crutches, weight bearing as tolerated, today. Clinic policy states that patients must be able to produce an active quadriceps femoris contraction prior to crutch-walking instruction. However, the patient is unable to produce an active contraction of the quadriceps femoris muscle. There is minimal pain and swelling, but after working with the patient for 15 minutes, he remains unable to contract the quadriceps femoris.

Impression: Status-post arthroscopic surgery on the right knee with inhibition of quadriceps femoris control.

Treatment Plan: Using a pulsatile monophasic waveform generator, a course of electrical stimulation was initiated. The cathode (active, negative polarity) was placed over the motor point of the vastus medialis, and the anode (inactive, positive polarity) was placed on the posterior thigh. The frequency was set at 40 pps. Using an uninterrupted (1:0) duty cycle, the amplitude was set to a level that produced a visible contraction, but was below the pain threshold. After establishing the stimulus amplitude, the duty cycle was then adjusted to deliver 15 seconds of stimulus followed by 15 seconds of rest; the current was not ramped, so the effective duty cycle was 1:1. The patient was encouraged to contract the quadriceps femoris during the stimulation for the first 5 stimulations, then was asked to contract the quadriceps femoris before the stimulus was delivered.

Response: After 20 repetitions of the stimulus, the patient was able to initiate a contraction of the quadriceps femoris before the current was delivered. The electrical stimulation was discontinued, and the patient was able to continue to contract the quadriceps femoris voluntarily. He was then instructed in crutch walking, and routine post-operative rehabilitation was initiated.

Case Study #2: ELECTRICAL STIMULATION: MUSCLE REEDUCATION

Background: A 23-year-old man experienced a Sunderland Grade V lesion of the left radial nerve as a result of an open fracture of the humerus sustained in a motorcycle accident. The injury occurred two years ago. There was an unsuccessful primary repair of the nerve injury; because there was no evidence of reinnervation, a sural nerve graft was completed one year ago. Again, there was no evidence of reinnervation, so the distal attachment of the flexor carpi radialis (FCR) was transferred to the posterior aspect of the base of the third metacarpal to provide wrist extension. The tendon transfer was completed three weeks ago. The wrist and forearm have been immobilized until yesterday, and the patient has been referred for rehabilitation. The surgeon has cleared the patient for gentle FCR contraction.

Impression: Post-tendon transfer with lack of voluntary control.

Treatment Plan: Using a pulsatile biphasic waveform generator, a course of therapeutic electrical stimulation was initiated. A bipolar electrode arrangement was used, with one electrode over the motor point of the FCR and the other electrode approximately four centimeters distal, over the FCR. The pulse rate was set at 40 pps, and the effective duty cycle was set at 5:5 (5 seconds on, 5 seconds off), with a 2 second ramp up and a 2 second ramp down (so the total time the current was delivered was 7 seconds, with 7 seconds between stimulations). The current amplitude was adjusted to achieve a palpable contraction of the FCR, but no wrist motion, and the treatment time was set to 12 minutes, so as to achieve approximately 50 contractions.

Response: Treatment was conducted daily for three weeks, with gradual increases in the current amplitude and number of repetitions. At this time, the patient was able to initiate wrist extension independent of the electrical stimulation, and was discharged to a home program.

Discussion Questions for Case Studies
*   What tissues were injured/affected?
*   What symptoms were present?
*   What phase of the injury-healing continuum did the patient present for care in?
*   What are the physical agent modality's biophysical effects? (direct/indirect/depth/tissue affinity)
*   What are the physical agent modality's indications/contraindications?
*   What are the parameters of the physical agent modality's application/dosage/duration/frequency in this case study?

The rehabilitation professional employs physical agent modalities to create an optimum environment for tissue healing while minimizing the symptoms associated with the trauma or condition.

What other physical agent modalities could be utilized to treat this injury or condition? Why? How?

Further Discussion Questions

- Why was the patient unable to contract the quadriceps femoris following surgery?

- Why was the ability to contract the quadriceps femoris a pre-requisite to crutch ambulation?

- What is the difference (pathway and physiology) between the voluntary muscle contraction and the induced (stimulated) contraction?

- How did the electrical stimulation assist the patient in regaining the ability to voluntarily contract the muscle?

- What is a viable alternative approach to assisting this patient?

- What would you suspect if there were no responses to the electrical stimulation?

- Why was the amplitude of stimulus set below the pain threshold?

- What structures are involved with a Sunderland Grade V peripheral nerve injury?

- What is involved in a sural nerve graft? What was the surgeon trying to achieve?

- What factors led to the failure of the primary radial nerve repair and the sural graft?

- Why did the surgeon wait nearly a year after the primary repair to do the sural graft, and nearly a year after the sural graft to perform the tendon transfer?

- Will wrist extension in the absence of extensor digitorum communis function really increase the patient's function? Why or why not?

ELECTRICAL STIMULATION: MUSCLE STRENGTHENING

DESCRIPTION:

Electrical stimulation is often used for increasing skeletal muscle strength (isometric force development capacity) by itself or in conjunction with active exercise. However, there is no evidence the electrical stimulation by itself or in conjunction with active exercise is better than active exercise alone for muscle strengthening. Also, the increase in tension developing capacity does not transfer to functional activities. Because of this, it is sometimes referred to as "electrical stimulation to increase isometric force development capacity".

PHYSIOLOGICAL EFFECTS:

- Depolarization of peripheral nerves

THERAPEUTIC EFFECTS:

- Increase in isometric force development capacity

INDICATIONS:

The primary indication is muscle weakness. However, electrical stimulation is sometimes used in an attempt to prevent disuse atrophy during immobilization of a limb.

CONTRAINDICATIONS:

- Pregnancy
- Implanted electrical pacing devices (e.g., cardiac pacemaker, bladder stimulator, etc.)
- Cardiac arrhythmia
- Over the carotid sinus area
- Hypersensitivity (i.e., the patient who has a strong aversion to electricity, or the patient with certain types of catheters or shunts).

ELECTRICAL STIMULATION: MUSCLE STRENGTHENING

PROCEDURE	Evaluation #		
	1	2	3
1. Check supplies			
a. Obtain towels or sheets for draping, conductant.			
b. Check stimulator, electrodes, and cables for charged battery, broken or frayed insulation, etc.			
c. Verify that the intensity control is at zero.			
2. Question patient			
a. Verify identity of patient (if not already verified).			
b. Verify the absence of contraindications.			
c. Ask about previous exposure to electrotherapy, check treatment notes.			
3. Position patient			
a. Place patient in a well-supported, comfortable position.			
b. Expose body part to be treated.			
c. Drape patient to preserve patient's modesty, protect clothing, but allow access to body part.			
4. Inspect body part to be treated			
a. Check light touch perception.			
b. Assess function of body part (e.g., ROM, irritability).			

Checklist continues

28

PROCEDURE	Evaluation #		
	1	2	3
5. Apply electrical stimulation for muscle strengthening			
a. Place conductant on electrodes as indicated, secure electrodes to patient. Electrode location will vary depending on desired effect. Usually, the ideal location for the active electrode is over the motor point of the target muscle, or the peripheral nerve trunk that supplies the target muscle.			
b. Remind the patient to inform you when they feel something. Do not tell the patient what they will feel; e.g., do not say "tell me when you feel a buzz or tingle."			
c. Adjust the pulse rate, pulse width, and mode of stimulation to desired settings if possible.			
d. Turn on the stimulator, and increase the amplitude slowly. Monitor the patient's response, not the stimulator.			
e. After the patient reports the onset of the stimulus, adjust the amplitude to as high a level as the patient can tolerate.			
f. Set a timer for the appropriate treatment time and give the patient a signaling device. Make sure the patient understands how to use the signaling device.			
g. Recheck the patient after about five minutes. If the sensation has diminished, adjust the amplitude appropriately.			

Checklist continues

PROCEDURE	Evaluation #		
	1	2	3
6. Complete treatment			
a. When the treatment time is over, turn the intensity control to zero, move the generator away from the patient; remove conductant with a towel.			
b. Remove material used for draping, assist the patient in dressing as needed.			
c. Have the patient perform appropriate therapeutic exercise as indicated.			
d. Clean the treatment area and equipment according to normal protocol.			
7. Assess treatment efficacy			
a. Ask the patient how the treated area feels.			
b. Visually inspect the treated area for any adverse reactions.			
c. Perform functional tests as indicated.			

CASE STUDY #1: ELECTRICAL STIMULATION: MUSCLE STRENGTHENING

Background: A 22-year-old female competitive soccer player sustained a severe grade II medial collateral ligament sprain of the left knee 3 days ago, and is being treated with plaster immobilization for 3 weeks. She is not able to generate a maximal isometric quadriceps contraction voluntarily. The cast has been modified to accommodate electrodes over the femoral nerve and the motor point of the vastus medialis muscle. There are no restrictions on the amount of force she is allowed to produce during a knee extension effort.

Impression: Grade II MCL sprain of the left knee, with inability to generate maximal isometric force of the knee extensors.

Treatment Plan: A five-day per week schedule of electrical stimulation was initiated. A polyphasic waveform was selected, with a 2500 Hz carrier wave, with an effective frequency of 50 Hz (10 ms on, 10 ms off). The stimulator was set to ramp the current up for 6 seconds, then maintain the current at a specific amplitude for 10 seconds, then drop to zero with no ramp; rest time was 50 seconds, giving an effective duty cycle of 1:5 (10 seconds on, 50 seconds off). Each treatment session began with 10 repetitions at comfortable stimulus amplitude, followed by 3 sets of 10 repetitions each with the maximal amount of current tolerable. A 2-minute rest separated the sets. During the 10 seconds on time, the current amplitude was adjusted to the maximal amount the patient was able to tolerate. The patient was encouraged to contract the quadriceps femoris muscle group as the current was delivered.

Response: The patient's tolerance for the electrical stimulation gradually increased during the first week, then reached a plateau; this plateau was maintained for the next two weeks. Upon removal of the cast, there was no measurable or visible atrophy of the left thigh. A rehabilitation program of active range of motion, strengthening exercise, and functional activities was initiated, and the patient returned to competition 2 weeks following cast removal.

Case Study #2: ELECTRICAL STIMULATION: MUSCLE STRENGTHENING

Background: A 33-year-old woman sustained an isolated rupture of the left anterior cruciate ligament (ACL) two weeks ago while skiing. Three days ago, she underwent an arthroscopically assisted intra-articular reconstruction of the ACL using an autologous patellar-ligament graft. She is now weight bearing as tolerated with axillary crutches, is using a removable splint, and has been cleared for accelerated rehabilitation.

Impression: Post-operative ACL reconstruction.

Treatment Plan: In addition to the standard active strengthening and range of motion exercise and physical agent modalities to control post-operative pain and swelling, a course of electrical stimulation for strengthening was initiated. The split was removed, and the patient was seated on an isokinetic testing and training device, with the left knee in 65 degrees of flexion, and the device set at a speed of 0 degrees per second (isometric). A pulsatile polyphasic electrical stimulator was used, with electrodes placed over the motor points of the vastus medialis and vastus lateralis muscles. The stimulator produced a 2500-Hz carrier wave, with an effective frequency of 50 Hz (10 msec on, 10 msec off). A two second ramp-up and a two second ramp-down setting was selected, with a total duty cycle of 10:50 (so 14 seconds on, 50 seconds off), and the current amplitude was adjusted to maximal tolerance during every third stimulation. Fifteen cycles were administered, then the patient rested for five minutes; this was repeated twice, for a total of 45 contractions per treatment session. The patient was treated three times per week for a total of five weeks.

Response: A linear increase in force produced during electrical stimulation, as well as maximal isometric force production, was recorded over the five weeks of treatment. The patient's gait and range of motion improved, and she was discharged to a home program at the end of treatment.

Discussion Questions for Case Studies

- What tissues were injured/affected?
- What symptoms were present?
- What phase of the injury-healing continuum did the patient present for care in?
- What are the physical agent modality's biophysical effects? (direct/indirect/depth/tissue affinity)
- What are the physical agent modality's indications/contraindications?
- What are the parameters of the physical agent modality's application/dosage/duration/frequency in this case study?

The rehabilitation professional employs physical agent modalities to create an optimum environment for tissue healing while minimizing the symptoms associated with the trauma or condition.

What other physical agent modalities could be utilized to treat this injury or condition? Why? How?

Further Discussion Questions

- Why was the adjective "severe" used with the phrase "Grade II sprain"?

- What tissues besides the MCL were likely affected by the injury?

- If the patient had performed a maximal isometric contraction of the left knee extensors the day after cast removal, what would you anticipate the force production to be compared to the right knee extensors? The left knee extensors prior to the injury?

- Is it probable that the electrical stimulation contributed to the patient's early return to competition? Could the electrical stimulation hasten the healing of the sprain?

- What advantages are there to augmenting the ACL repair with the patellar tendon?

- Why was the training of the quadriceps femoris conducted at 65 degrees of flexion? What biomechanical factors favor training at this joint angle as opposed to full extension of the knee?

- What effect did the electrical stimulation have on the healing rate of the reconstruction? On the patient's return to function?

ELECTRICAL STIMULATION: IONTOPHORESIS

DESCRIPTION:

     Iontophoresis is the use of direct current electricity to introduce various drugs to subcutaneous tissues without using invasive means. Though there are many drugs that may be used, various corticosterioids and local anesthetics are the most commonly used drugs.

     It is not possible to use any form of electrical current other than direct current to achieve movement of the drug; the misnamed "high voltage galvanic stimulators" are not capable of phoresing a drug due to the very low pulse charge. Because of the possibility of producing an electrolytic burn with direct current, it is recommended that the current amplitude remain below $0.7 \text{ mA} \cdot \text{cm}^{-2}$ of electrode.

     There are many different electrodes available for iontophoresis. The most rudimentary is to use alligator clips to attach the cables to a tin or aluminum conductor, and use a paper towel soaked with the drug between the electrode and the patient. More commonly, electrodes developed by the manufacturer of the stimulator are used.

     It is mandatory that the drug is in an ionic form; otherwise, the electrical current will not be able to move the drug. Many drugs come in both ionized forms and as a suspension. If in doubt, a PDR should be consulted.

PHYSIOLOGICAL EFFECTS:
* Depends on the drug

THERAPEUTIC EFFECTS:
* Depends on the drug; generally, decreased inflammation and local anesthesia

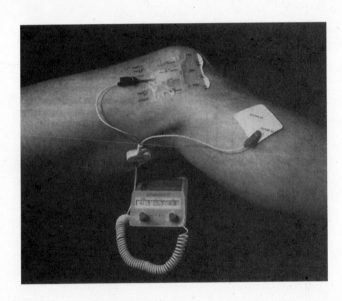

INDICATIONS:

The primary indication is for the treatment of superficial soft and connective tissue inflammations involving muscle, tendon, ligament, capsule and integument.

CONTRAINDICATIONS:
- Pregnancy
- Implanted electrical pacing devices (e.g., cardiac pacemaker, bladder stimulator, etc.)
- Cardiac arrhythmia
- Over the carotid sinus area
- Hypersensitivity (i.e., the patient who has a strong aversion to electricity, or the patient with certain types of catheters or shunts) or known drug allergy.

ELECTRICAL STIMULATION: IONTOPHORESIS

PROCEDURE	Evaluation #		
	1	2	3
1. Check supplies			
a. Obtain towels or sheets for draping, conductant.			
b. Check stimulator, electrodes, and cables for charged battery, broken or frayed insulation, etc.			
c. Verify that the intensity control is at zero.			
2. Question patient			
a. Verify identity of patient (if not already verified).			
b. Verify the absence of contraindications.			
c. Ask about previous exposure to electrotherapy.			
3. Position patient			
a. Place patient in a well-supported, comfortable position.			
b. Expose body part to be treated.			
c. Drape patient to preserve patient's modesty, protect clothing, but allow access to body part.			
4. Inspect body part to be treated			
a. Check light touch perception.			
b. Assess function of body part (e.g., ROM, irritability)			
5. Apply electrical stimulation for iontophoresis			
a. Prepare electrodes according to manufacturer's instructions, secure electrodes to patient. Electrode location will vary depending on the drug being phoresed; anionic drugs are repelled from the cathode, cations are repelled from the anode.			

Checklist continues

36

PROCEDURE	Evaluation #		
	1	2	3
b. Remind the patient to inform you when they feel something. Do not tell the patient what they will feel; e.g., do not say "tell me when you feel a burning or stinging."			
c. Turn on the stimulator, and increase the amplitude slowly. Monitor the patient's response, not the stimulator.			
d. After the patient reports the onset of the stimulus, adjust the amplitude to the appropriate intensity.			
e. Continue to monitor the patient during the duration of the treatment.			
6. Complete treatment			
a. When the treatment time is over, turn the generator off, and turn the intensity control to zero; remove conductant with a towel.			
b. Remove material used for draping, assist the patient in dressing as needed.			
c. Have the patient perform appropriate therapeutic exercise as indicated.			
d. Clean the treatment area and equipment according to normal protocol.			
7. Assess treatment efficacy			
a. Ask the patient how the treated area feels.			
b. Visually inspect the treated area for any adverse reactions.			
c. Perform functional tests as indicated.			

Case Study #1: ELECTRICAL STIMULATION - IONTOPHORESIS

Background: A 48-year-old man developed pain in the region inferior to the right patella subsequent to a fall onto the knee while playing tennis. There was immediate mild, localized swelling, which resolved with ice and rest. The acute pain subsided after about 7 days, but the patient then noted significant stiffness following rest, localized tenderness, and pain with climbing stairs, squatting, and kneeling. The physical examination was benign except for mild swelling and point tenderness of the infrapatellar tendon, as well as creptius to palpation of the tendon during active knee extension.

Impression: Infrapatellar tendinitis.

Treatment Plan: In addition to rest and local ice application, a course of iontophoresis of dexamethasone was initiated. The area was prepared appropriately, and the cathode (negative polarity) was used as the delivery electrode. A total of 60 milliamp (min of current) was delivered on an every-other-day schedule for a total of six treatments.

Response: There was a slight increase in the symptoms following the initial treatment, which persisted for approximately 12 hours following the second treatment. The signs and symptoms then began to diminish, and the patient was symptom-free following the fifth treatment. A progressive increase in physical activity was initiated, and the patient returned to pre-injury function four weeks later.

Case Study #2: ELECTRICAL STIMULATION - IONTOPHORESIS

Background: A 28-year-old woman has a three-week history of bilateral wrist pain and nocturnal paresthesia in the palmar aspect of the thumb, index, and long fingers. The symptoms started two weeks after starting a new job working on the trim line of an automobile manufacturing plant. The job involves repetitive motions with both hands, and a great deal of squeezing to seat weather-stripping in the doors. The paresthesia is provoked with driving, holding the telephone, and a blow dryer. She has pain with passive wrist and finger extension and resisted finger flexion, and paresthesia is produced with compression over the carpal tunnel for 15 seconds. She has a positive Tinel sign over the median nerve at the distal wrist crease, and a positive Phalen test at 30 seconds. Crepitus is noted on the anterior wrist with finger flexion.

Impression: Tenosynovitis of the flexor digitorum tendons, with acute carpal tunnel syndrome.

Treatment Plan: The patient was instructed to use resting hand splints at night, and a course of iontophoresis was initiated for the right wrist only. In addition, work restrictions were placed on the patient, to avoid repetitive motion and gripping activities. Dexamethasone was delivered from the cathode (negative polarity), which was placed over the carpal tunnel, with the anode placed over the dorsum of the wrist. A total of 45 milliamp minutes of current were delivered three days per week for two weeks.

Response: The patient's symptoms diminished in both hands over the two-week period; however, she continued to have a positive carpal compression test, a positive Phalen test, and a positive Tinel sign only on the left. She returned to the trim line with instructions for a two-week ramp-up period; however, the pain and paresthesia returned in the left wrist. She was subsequently treated with iontophoresis on the left wrist, and was able to return to work without restrictions following a second two-week ramp-up period.

Discussion Questions for Case Studies

- What tissues were injured/affected?
- What symptoms were present?
- What phase of the injury-healing continuum did the patient present for care in?
- What are the physical agent modality's biophysical effects? (direct/indirect/depth/tissue affinity)
- What are the physical agent modality's indications/contraindications?
- What are the parameters of the physical agent modality's application/dosage/duration/ frequency in this case study?

The rehabilitation professional employs physical agent modalities to create an optimum environment for tissue healing while minimizing the symptoms associated with the trauma or condition.

What other physical agent modalities could be utilized to treat this injury or condition? Why? How?

Further Discussion Questions

- What is the pathophysiology of tendinitis?

- What is the mechanism of action of the dexamethasone?

- What is the polarity of the dexamethasone molecule?

- What are the required and ideal characteristics for a molecule to be introduced via iontophoresis?

- What are the advantages and disadvantages of iontophoresis as compared to a needle injection?

- Why did the symptoms increase initially?

- What is the significance of the Tinel sign?

- What is the significance of the Phalen test?

- Why does compression over the carpal tunnel reproduce the symptoms?

- Why does the patient experience nocturnal paresthesia rather than during work?

- What is another potential source of the patient's symptoms?

- If the patient also had cervical pain, would you anticipate a different treatment approach?

- Would electrophysiologic testing be appropriate for this patient?

Chapter 4: BIOFEEDBACK

DESCRIPTION:

Biofeedback utilizes the body's self-generated motor unit action potentials (MUAP). These signals are recorded by surface electrodes, amplified then processed and converted into audio or visual signals to allow an individual to monitor various psychophysiological processes and recognize appropriate responses.

PHYSIOLOGICAL EFFECTS:

- Increase level of motor unit activation
- Decrease level of motor unit activation

THERAPEUTIC EFFECTS:

- Increase Level of Muscle Activation (Muscle Reeducation)
- Decrease Level of Muscle Activation (Reduce Spasticity)
- General Body Muscular Relaxation

INDICATIONS:

Biofeedback is primarily employed by the sports therapist as an adjunct in the reeducation of muscle function following injury, immobilization or surgery or as an aid to identifying unwanted levels of muscle activity (spasticity) which may be interfering with the athlete's recovery. Sometimes biofeedback is used as a tool to assess the body's general neuromuscular status as an aid in relaxation to reduce pain and/or anxiety.

CONTRAINDICATIONS:

- Possible Skin Irritation at Electrode Site From Coupling Gel or Adhesives

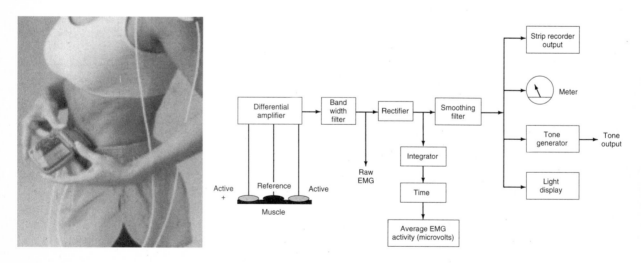

BIOFEEDBACK

PROCEDURE	Evaluation #		
	1	2	3
1. Check Supplies			
a. Obtain biofeedback unit, coupling gel and tape			
b. Insure that batteries in unit are fresh			
2. Question Patient			
a. Verify identity of patient and review previous treatment notes			
b. Verify the absence of contraindications			
3. Position Patient			
a. Place patient in a well-supported, comfortable position			
b. Select and expose appropriate muscle/group to monitor			
c. Drape patient to preserve patient's modesty, protect clothing, but allow access to muscle/group			
4. Select appropriate electrode			
5. Prepare the electrode site			
a. Clean the skin surface with alcohol or soap and water			
6. Apply the electrodes			
a. Secure with tape or wrap			
7. Explain the procedure to patient			
8. Begin the indicated procedure			
a. Muscle Reeducation			
1. Adjust unit to lowest threshold (uV's) that picks up any activity (MUAP's)			
2. Adjust audio/visual feedback			

Checklist continues

3. Have patient contract target muscle to produce maximum audio/visual feedback			
4. Facilitate target muscle contraction as necessary by tapping, stroking or contracting opposite like muscle			
5. When maximum feedback is obtained for selected threshold advance threshold and attempt again			
6. Advance muscle/limb to other positions			
7. Continue muscle contractions for 10 - 15 minutes per training session or until maximal muscle activation is obtained			
b. Spasticity Inhibition			
1. Adjust unit to sensitivity threshold (uV's) that picks up maximal activity (MUAP's)			
2. Adjust audio/visual feedback			
3. Have patient relax target muscle to produce minimum audio/visual feedback			
4. Facilitate target muscle relaxation as necessary by tapping, stroking or contracting opposite like muscle			
5. When minimum feedback is obtained for selected threshold reduce threshold and attempt relaxation again			
6. Advance muscle/limb to other functional positions			
7. Continue muscle relaxation for 10 - 15 minutes per training session or until muscle relaxation is obtained			

Checklist continues

8.	Complete the treatment.			
	a. Remove the electrodes			
	b. Clean electrode site			
	c. Record results of session			
	d. Assess treatment efficacy			
9.	Instruct the patient in any indicated exercise			
10.	Return Equipment to Storage After Cleaning			

Case Study #1: BIOFEEDBACK

Background: A 14 year old female subluxed her left patella while at soccer practice. There was immediate pain and a localized effusion, which resolved with the use of an immobilizer, intermittent ice packs and rest over a seven-day period. Upon referral for the initiation of quadriceps rehabilitation the patient reported no pain, minimal swelling but residual stiffness and sensation of weakness in the knee joint. The physical examination was unremarkable except for limited ROM of 10 -110 degrees and the inability of the patient to successfully initiate and sustain an isometric contraction of the quadriceps musculature.

Impression: Quadriceps inhibition secondary to injury and immobilization.

Treatment Plan: In addition to the initiation of therapeutic exercise - static stretching and active-assistive ROM exercise for the knee joint; biofeedback was initiated for the quadriceps mechanism. Using the vastus medialis muscle as the target muscle, the skin was cleansed and electrodes placed in alignment with the fibers of the muscle. A microvolt threshold of detection slightly above the patient's ability to maximize auditory and visual feedback was chosen. The patient was encouraged to perform isometric quadriceps setting exercises of 6 - 10 seconds duration attempting to "max out" feedback for the chosen threshold level. The threshold was advanced and the process repeated.

Response: Over the course of the initial rehabilitation session, the patient advanced several threshold levels and "reacquired" the ability to initiate and sustain an isometric quadriceps muscle contraction comparable to her uninvolved extremity. She was rapidly transitioned to limited range dynamic exercise and a functional closed-chain exercise sequence with emphasis on terminal range knee stability. She returned to soccer activities several weeks later.

Case Study #2: BIOFEEDBACK

Background: A 19-year-old male suffered a twisting injury to the right knee during football practice. There was immediate pain, effusion, joint line tenderness and hamstring muscle spasm that prevented full extension of the knee. Initial treatment involved the use of an immobilizer, intermittent application of ice packs, elevation and rest over the first 24 hours post-injury. Referral for rehabilitation was immediate and the patient reported to the clinic with residual pain, minimal swelling but with residual hamstring muscle guarding which prevented full active or passive knee extension.

Impression: Hamstring muscle spasm secondary to injury.

Treatment Plan: Therapeutic exercise – PNF contract – relax was initiated for the knee joint musculature – primarily the hamstrings; biofeedback was also initiated for the hamstring muscles.

Using the semimembranosus/semitendinosus muscles as the targets, the skin was cleansed and electrodes placed in alignment with the fibers of the muscles. A microvolt threshold of detection at the level of the patient's current muscle spasm activity was chosen with continuous auditory feedback. The patient was encouraged to isometrically contract his hamstring muscles, and then consciously think of relaxing the muscles and reducing the level of auditory feedback. When auditory silence was achieved for the chosen microvolt level, the threshold was reduced and the process repeated. The patient was then encouraged to actively and passively extend the knee.

Response: Over the course of the initial rehabilitation session, the patient was able to reduce the threshold level and "relax" the hamstring muscles to achieve full active and passive knee extension comparable to his uninvolved extremity. He was rapidly transitioned to dynamic exercise and a functional closed -chain exercise sequence with emphasis on terminal range knee stability. He returned to football activities several weeks later.

Discussion Questions
- What tissues were injured/affected?
- What symptoms were present?
- What phase of the injury-healing continuum did the patient present for care in?
- What are the physical agent modality's biophysical effects? (direct/indirect/depth/tissue affinity)
- What are the physical agent modality's indications/contraindications?
- What are the parameters of the physical agent modality's application/dosage/duration/ frequency in this case study?

The rehabilitation professional employs physical agent modalities to create an optimum environment for tissue healing while minimizing the symptoms associated with the trauma or condition.

What other physical agent modalities could be utilized to treat this injury or condition? Why? How?

Further Discussion Questions

- How would biofeedback assist in this patient's course of rehabilitation?

- How did the biofeedback assist the patient's muscle contraction effort?

- What would the goal of each treatment session be?

- How long would you continue the use of biofeedback with this patient? What objective criteria could you use?

- Describe how you would integrate PNF techniques with Biofeedback.

Chapter 5: SHORTWAVE DIATHERMY

DESCRIPTION:

Shortwave diathermy (SWD; diathermy means to heat through) utilizes an alternating current (most commonly 27.12 Mhz) passed either through a coiled conductor or to a capacitor plate. With the coil method, the patient is placed in the magnetic field that is generated when the current passes through the coil; the magnetic field then is absorbed by the molecules in the body, increasing their internal energy. This method is referred to as inductive, because the body acts as a secondary coil, and the current in the body is induced by the current in the primary coil; the body never becomes part of the electrical circuit. With the second method, there are two capacitor plates that are charged, and the body acts as a lower resistance conductor for the discharge of the capacitive current; thus the term capacitive short wave diathermy. Again, the molecules of the body absorb the energy, and have their internal energy increased. In capacitive SWD, the patient becomes part of the electrical circuit.

Because the motion of a molecule is dependent upon it's internal energy, when a molecule absorbs any type of energy, it's motion increases. Temperature is a reflection of the average kinetic energy of a system, and the kinetic energy is by definition the random molecular motion. Therefore, when the molecular motion increases, the temperature increases. Although there are increased molecular collisions when the thermal energy of a system increases, these collisions do not produce any energy; they merely transfer the energy from one molecule to another. It is a misconception that the "friction" that occurs between the molecules causes the increased temperature.

Although electrical energy is used in SWD, action potentials are not induced in excitable tissue. At such high frequencies, the phase charge of the current is inadequate to alter the membrane voltage enough for the membrane to reach threshold. The amount of heat generated does follow Joule's law, where $Q = I^2Rt$, with Q being heat, I being current, R resistance, and t time. The heat is generated in the tissue that absorbs the energy, and this varies according to the type of SWD used. Inductive SWD is absorbed mostly by tissues that have a high electrical conductivity, such as muscle. Capacitive SWD is absorbed mostly by tissues that have a low electrical conductivity, such as skin and fat. Because of this, capacitive SWD does not penetrate as deeply as inductive SWD, but does produce a more marked sensation of warmth in the patient. The general guideline for the depth of penetration of capacitive SWD is one centimeter, and three to four centimeters for inductive SWD.

PHYSIOLOGICAL EFFECTS:

- Vasodilation
- Decreased pain perception
- Increased local metabolism
- Increased connective tissue plasticity
- Decreased isometric strength (transient)

THERAPEUTIC EFFECTS:

- Decreased pain
- Increased soft tissue extensibility

INDICATIONS:

Shortwave diathermy is a heating physical agent; therefore, the indications are the same as for any heating agent. However, the depth of penetration, at least for inductive SWD, is greater than for any of the infrared agents. Ultrasound has a deeper penetration than SWD, but SWD can be used to treat a much larger area.

CONTRAINDICATIONS:

- Lack of normal temperature sensibility
- Peripheral vascular disease with compromised circulation
- Over tumors, the testes, open growth plates, acutely inflamed tissue, active hemorrhage, the eyes, or metallic objects
- Pregnancy
- In patients with implanted electrical stimulators (e.g., cardiac pacemakers, phrenic nerve stimulators, etc.)

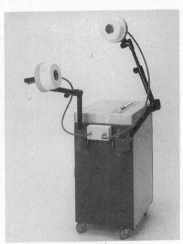

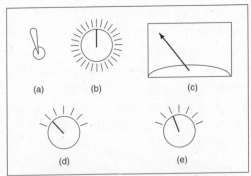

(a) (b) (c)

(d) (e)

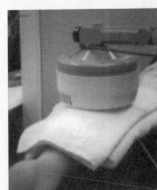

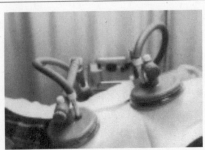

SHORTWAVE DIATHERMY

PROCEDURE	Evaluation #		
	1	2	3
1. Check supplies			
a. Obtain sheet or towels for draping, timer, signaling device.			
b. Check SWD generator for frayed power cords, integrity cables and drum, shields, etc.			
c. Verify that the output control is at zero.			
2. Question patient			
a. Verify identity of patient (if not already verified).			
b. Verify the absence of contraindications.			
c. Ask about previous thermotherapy treatments, check treatment notes.			
3. Position patient			
a. Place patient in a well-supported, comfortable position. This is particularly crucial, because the patient should not shift positions after the treatment starts.			
b. Expose body part to be treated, have patient remove all jewelry from the area.			
c. Drape patient to preserve patient's modesty, protect clothing, but allow access to body part.			
4. Inspect body part to be treated			
a. Check light touch perception.			
b. Check circulatory status (pulses, capillary refill).			

Checklist continues

PROCEDURE	Evaluation #		
	1	2	3
c. Assess function of body part (e.g., ROM, irritability).			
5. Apply SWD			
a. Place a single layer of towel on the treatment area.			
b. **Inductive**: position the drum containing the coil parallel to the body part and in contact with the towel. (Figure 5-1). **Capacitive**: position the plates parallel to the body part and about 2.5 to 7.5 centimeters away from the body. (Figure 5-2).			
c. Turn on the SWD generator, allow to warm up if necessary.			
d. Inform the patient that they should feel only warmth; if it becomes hot, they should inform you immediately.			
e. Adjust intensity of SWD to the appropriate level. Set a timer for the appropriate treatment time and give the patient a signaling device. Make sure the patient understands how to use the signaling device.			
f. Check the patient's response after the first five minutes by asking the patient how it feels. Recheck verbally about every 5 minutes.			

Checklist continues

PROCEDURE	Evaluation #		
	1	2	3
6. Complete the treatment			
a. When the treatment time is over, turn the intensity control to zero, and move the generator away from the patient; dry the area with a towel.			
b. Remove material used for draping, assist the patient in dressing as needed.			
c. Have the patient perform appropriate therapeutic exercise as indicated.			
d. Clean the treatment area and equipment according to normal protocol.			
7. Assess treatment efficacy			
a. Ask the patient how the treated area feels.			
b. Visually inspect the treated area for any adverse reactions.			
c. Perform functional tests as indicated.			

Case Study #1: SHORTWAVE DIATHERMY

Background: A thirty-two year old graduate student developed the gradual onset of lumbar paravertebral muscle spasm following a self-made move of her apartment contents. The symptoms were noted the day after the move upon arising and were described as a tightness and restriction of mobility in the low back. She reported no radiation of her symptoms into the buttocks or legs and no difficulty with bowel or bladder function. Physical examination revealed restriction in forward flexion and side rotation of the trunk with tenderness to palpation in the lumbar paravertebral musculature one week after the extensive bending and lifting.

Impression: Lumbar paravertebral muscle strain, sub acute

Treatment Plan: The patient was initiated on a course of inductive short wave diathermy to the lumbar paravertebral musculature, followed by active and active-assisted lumbar region range of motion exercise. Treatment was provided on an every other day basis for two weeks with increasing emphasis on mobilizing and strengthening the lumbar paravertebral musculature.

Response: The patient experienced immediate, but short duration relief of her low back pain following the initial treatment and enthusiastically pursued her exercise sequence. With each subsequent session, the duration of relief and improved trunk mobility increased. At the two week point in the treatment regimen the patient was independent in the performance of her lumbar exercise regimen and scheduled to attend a back education class prior to discharge.

Case Study #2: SHORTWAVE DIATHERMY

Background: A 53-year-old recreational athlete with documented osteoarthritis of the right knee comes to your clinic with a history of increasing pain and swelling over the past two months, coincident with an increased frequency of playing tennis. Because of the pain and swelling, he has developed a remarkable gait deviation, and is beginning to note more quadriceps atrophy. He was referred for quadriceps strengthening exercises, joint protection activities, and gait training as appropriate.

Impression: Degenerative joint disease with concurrent muscle inhibition and atrophy.

Treatment Plan: The patient received 15 minutes of capacitive shortwave diathermy prior to initiating quadriceps exercise. He reported short-term relief, which allowed the performance of his exercise program. Treatment was provided twice per week, with the patient given specific instructions in the performance of home lower member closed-chain exercises two times per week.

Response: At the tenth visit, the patient was discharged because of the ability to self-manage his condition. He continued to have mild post-tennis swelling and stiffness, minimal quadriceps atrophy, and a gait deviation only when very tired.

Discussion Questions for Case Studies

- What tissues were injured/affected?
- What symptoms were present?
- What phase of the injury-healing continuum did the patient present for care in?
- What are the physical agent modality's biophysical effects? (direct/indirect/depth/tissue affinity)
- What are the physical agent modality's indications/contraindications?
- What are the parameters of the physical agent modality's application/dosage/duration/ frequency in this case study?

The rehabilitation professional employs physical agent modalities to create an optimum environment for tissue healing while minimizing the symptoms associated with the trauma or condition.

What other physical agent modalities could be utilized to treat this injury or condition? Why? How?

Further Discussion Questions

- Was the choice of SWD optimal for this patient's suspected injury?
- What other things would you counsel this patient to be aware of while undergoing diathermy treatment?

Chapter 6: INFRARED PHYSICAL AGENTS

Thermotherapy - Hot Pack

DESCRIPTION:

Commercially available hot packs ("hydrocollator packs") are usually a canvas cover filled with a hydrophilic substance such as bentonite. Hot packs are kept in a commercial water-filled container that maintains a temperature of approximately 71° C (165-172 F). The packs are wrapped in six to eight layers of dry towels to protect the patient from burns; commercial hot pack covers provide approximately four thickness of toweling. After use, the hot pack should be returned to the cabinet for at least 30 minutes to insure re-heating. Hot packs provide only superficial heating; the maximum depth of therapeutic heating is only about one centimeter, and occurs within 10 minutes of application.

PHYSIOLOGICAL EFFECTS:

- Vasodilation
- Decreased pain perception
- Increased local metabolism
- Increased connective tissue plasticity
- Decreased isometric strength (transient)

THERAPEUTIC EFFECTS:

- Decreased pain
- Increased soft tissue extensibility

INDICATIONS:

The principal indication for a hot pack is to provide therapeutic warming of superficial tissues. Tissues that are deeper than one centimeter do not reach a therapeutic temperature range of $\geq 40°$ C. Therefore, if the target tissue is deeper than one centimeter (e.g., the spinal facet joints), a hot pack will not be effective. Other joints, such as the knee, wrist, and ankle, can be effectively heated with a hot pack.

The primary therapeutic effect of superficial heating is to increase the ability of the collagen to remodel. Therefore, heating the tissue is beneficial following a period of reduced mobility if the soft tissue has shortened. In addition, the tissue viscosity is reduced, resulting in a greater ease of motion through the available range of motion. Though generally not a problem, in case of extreme pressure sensitivity, the weight of a hot pack may be more than the patient can tolerate. In these cases, Fluidotherapy® or a warm whirlpool may be helpful.

CONTRAINDICATIONS:

- Lack of normal temperature sensibility
- Peripheral vascular disease with compromised circulation
- Over tumors

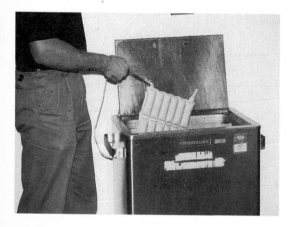
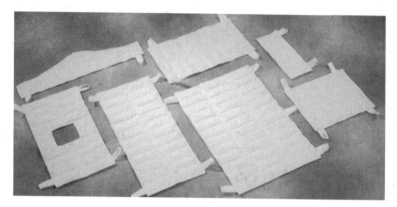
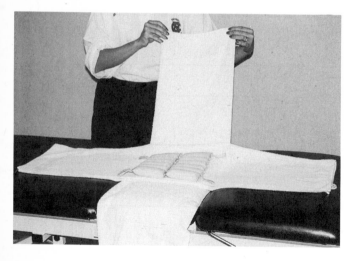
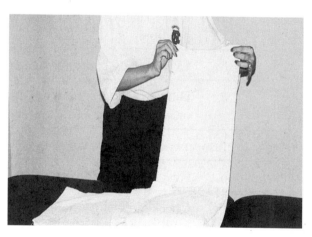

HOT PACK

PROCEDURE	Evaluation #		
	1	2	3
1. Check supplies			
a. Obtain dry towels to wrap hot pack in, sheet or towels for draping, timer, signaling device.			
b. Check appropriate temperature. Remove hot pack. (Figure 6-1)			
2. Question patient			
a. Verify identity of patient (if not already verified).			
b. Verify the absence of contraindications.			
c. Ask about previous thermotherapy treatments, check treatment notes.			
3. Position patient			
a. Place patient in a well-supported, comfortable position.			
b. Expose body part to be treated.			
c. Drape patient to preserve patient's modesty, protect clothing, but allow access to body part.			
4. Inspect body part to be treated			
a. Check light touch perception.			
b. Check circulatory status (pulses, capillary refill).			
c. Verify that there are no open wounds or rashes.			
d. Assess function of body part (e.g., ROM, irritability).			

Checklist continues

PROCEDURE	Evaluation #		
	1	2	3
5. Apply hot pack			
a. Wrap hot pack in towels to provide six to eight layers of towel between the hot pack and the patient. If using a commercial hot pack cover, use at least one layer of towel to keep the cover clean. (Figure 6-2)			
b. Inform the patient that you are going to put the hot pack on the body part to be treated, then do so.			
c. Set a timer for the appropriate treatment time and give the patient a signaling device. Make sure the patient understands how to use the signaling device.			
d. Check the patient's response after the first five minutes by asking the patient how it feels as well as visually checking the area under the hot pack. If the area is blotchy, additional toweling may be needed. Recheck verbally about every 5 minutes. A visual inspection every 5 minutes is not inappropriate.			

Checklist continues

PROCEDURE	Evaluation #		
	1	2	3
6. Complete the treatment			
a. When the treatment time is over, remove the hot pack and dry the area with a towel.			
b. Remove material used for draping, assist the patient in dressing as needed.			
c. Have the patient perform appropriate therapeutic exercise as indicated.			
d. Clean the treatment area and equipment according to normal protocol.			
7. Assess treatment efficacy			
a. Ask the patient how the treated area feels.			
b. Visually inspect the treated area for any adverse reactions.			
c. Perform functional tests as indicated.			

Case Study: THERMOTHERAPY - HOT PACK

Background: A 15-year-old boy sustained a non-comminuted, transverse fracture of the left patella during a football game 6 weeks ago. He was treated with plaster immobilization for 6 weeks; the cast was removed yesterday. He has full knee extension (the knee was immobilized in full extension), and has only 20 degrees of flexion. The patella is well healed and non-tender, and patellar mobility is severely limited. As an adjunct to active and passive exercise, you begin joint mobilization of the patello-femoral joint every day. To enhance the response of the connective tissue, you decide to increase the tissue temperature prior to mobilization.

Impression: Limitation of motion secondary to fracture and immobilization.

Treatment Plan: Because the target tissues are immediately sub-cutaneous, you elect to use a hydrocollator pack. Using a cervical pack, heat was applied to the circumference of the knee for 12 minutes. Immediately after removal of the hot pack, joint mobilization was initiated. Following joint mobilization, active range of motion and strengthening exercises were performed.

Response: The patient was treated 3 days per week for 4 weeks, then discharged to a home program. He had full active and passive range of motion, patellar mobility was normal, and strength was 80% of the unaffected limb.

Discussion Questions for Case Study

- What tissues were injured/affected?
- What symptoms were present?
- What phase of the injury-healing continuum did the patient present for care in?
- What are the physical agent modality's biophysical effects? (direct/indirect/depth/tissue affinity)
- What are the physical agent modality's indications/contraindications?
- What are the parameters of the physical agent modality's application/dosage/duration/ frequency in this case study?

The rehabilitation professional employs physical agent modalities to create an optimum environment for tissue healing while minimizing the symptoms associated with the trauma or condition.

What other physical agent modalities could be utilized to treat this injury or condition? Why? How?

Further Discussion Questions

- What is the mechanism of heat transfer in this case?
- What is the effective depth of penetration of the heat using a Hydrocollator Pack?
- If there had been a significant layer of adipose below the skin, would the physical agent modality selection be the same?
- What are the physiological effects of heat?
- What are the advantages and disadvantages of using a Hydrocollator Pack for this patient?
- What alternative methods would have achieved the same effect?

Thermotherapy - Paraffin Bath

DESCRIPTION:

Paraffin baths consist of dipping and removing or immersing the body part in a mixture of wax and mineral oil. The ratio of wax and mineral oil is about 7:1, which results in a substance with a melting point of about 47.8° C, a specific heat of about $0.65 \ cal \cdot g^{-1} \cdot °C^{-1}$, and a therapeutic temperature range of 48 to 54°C. Because of the low specific heat, much higher temperatures can be tolerated than if water is used. The paraffin is kept in a thermostatically controlled cabinet.

Paraffin provides a superficial heat, with a depth of therapeutic heating of about one centimeter. However, because paraffin is generally used only for the hands and feet, the depth of penetration is adequate to warm these joints to a therapeutic range.

The two basic techniques of application of paraffin involve repeated dipping of the body part in the mixture, then covering the body part with plastic and toweling. The advantage of this method is that the body part can then be elevated, reducing the potential for swelling. The second method involves dipping the body part in the paraffin once, letting it dry for a few seconds, then immersing the body part for the duration of the treatment. The advantage of this technique is that the source of heat is constant, so the therapeutic temperature can be maintained for a longer period.

PHYSIOLOGICAL EFFECTS:

- Vasodilation
- Decreased pain perception
- Increased local metabolism
- Increased connective tissue plasticity
- Decreased isometric strength (transient)

THERAPEUTIC EFFECTS:

- Decreased pain
- Increased soft tissue extensibility

INDICATIONS:

The principal indication for a paraffin bath is to provide therapeutic warming of superficial tissues. This is particularly effective in the hands and feet following a period of immobilization. The increased connective tissue plasticity that occurs with warming will enhance the effectiveness of therapeutic exercise.

Paraffin baths are also helpful in alleviation of pain due to arthritic changes in the hands and feet. Caution should be exercised in using paraffin (or any heating agent) during an acute phase of arthritic pain and swelling.

CONTRAINDICATIONS:

- Lack of normal temperature sensibility
- Peripheral vascular disease with compromised circulation
- Over tumors

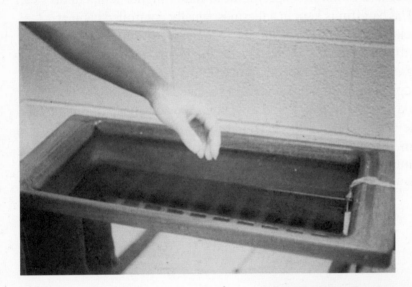

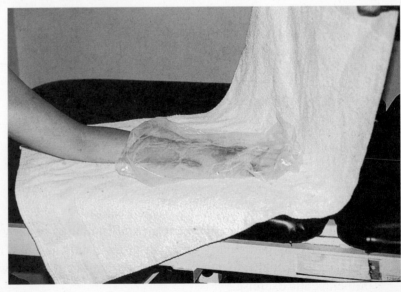

PARAFFIN BATH

PROCEDURE	Evaluation #		
	1	2	3
1. Check supplies			
a. Obtain plastic bag and towels to wrap body part in, timer, signaling device.			
b. Check cabinet for appropriate temperature.			
2. Question patient			
a. Verify identity of patient (if not already verified).			
b. Verify the absence of contraindications.			
c. Ask about previous thermotherapy treatments, check treatment notes.			
3. Prepare patient			
a. Have patient remove all jewelry from body part, wash well and dry thoroughly.			
b. Explain to the patient that after dipping the body part into the paraffin, there should be no movement of the body part for the duration of the treatment.			
4. Inspect body part to be treated			
a. Check light touch perception.			
b. Check circulatory status (pulses, capillary refill).			
c. Verify that there are no open wounds or rashes.			
d. Assess function of body part (e.g., ROM, irritability).			

Checklist continues

PROCEDURE	Evaluation #		
	1	2	3
5. Apply paraffin			
a. Guide the body part into the paraffin, making sure the patient does not contact the bottom of the cabinet or the heating coils. (Figure 6-3).			
b. After two or three seconds, remove the body part, and keep it above the paraffin so that none of the paraffin drips onto the floor. Re-immerse the body part, and repeat until the appropriate number of dips have been completed, or re-immerse for the duration of the treatment.			
c. Set a timer for the appropriate treatment time and give the patient a signaling device. Make sure the patient understands how to use the signaling device.			
d. Check the patient's response after the first five minutes by asking the patient how it feels. Recheck verbally about every 5 minutes.			

Checklist continues

PROCEDURE	Evaluation #		
	1	2	3
6. Complete the treatment			
a. When the treatment time is over, remove the towel and plastic bag. Help the patient remove the paraffin, and either return the paraffin to the cabinet, or throw away according to local protocol.			
b. Have the patient thoroughly wash and dry the body part.			
c. Have the patient perform appropriate therapeutic exercise as indicated.			
d. Clean the treatment area and equipment according to normal protocol.			
7. Assess treatment efficacy			
a. Ask the patient how the treated area feels.			
b. Visually inspect the treated area for any adverse reactions.			
c. Perform functional tests as indicated.			

Case Study: THERMOTHERAPY - PARAFFIN BATH

Background: A 14-year-old female softball catcher sustained a fracture of the distal phalanx of the ring finger on her throwing hand during a game 5 weeks ago. She was treated with immobilization for 5 weeks; the splint was removed yesterday. She had only 10 degrees of flexion at the DIP joint. The phalanx is well healed and non-tender. As an adjunct to active and passive exercise, you wish to begin joint mobilization. To enhance the response of the connective tissue, you decide to increase the tissue temperature prior to mobilization.

Impression: Limitation of motion secondary to fracture and immobilization.

Treatment Plan: Because the target tissues are immediately sub-cutaneous, you elect to use paraffin bath. Following standard protocol, paraffin was applied to the ring finger for 15 minutes. Immediately after removal of the paraffin, joint mobilization was initiated. Following joint mobilization, active range of motion and strengthening exercises were performed.

Response: The patient was treated 3 days per week for 2 weeks, then discharged to a home program. She had full active and passive range of motion, digit mobility was normal, and strength was sufficient for gripping and throwing.

Discussion Questions for Case Study

- What tissues were injured/affected?
- What symptoms were present?
- What phase of the injury-healing continuum did the patient present for care in?
- What are the physical agent modality's biophysical effects? (direct/indirect/depth/tissue affinity)
- What are the physical agent modality's indications/contraindications?
- What are the parameters of the physical agent modality's application/dosage/duration/ frequency in this case study?

     The rehabilitation professional employs physical agent modalities to create an optimum environment for tissue healing while minimizing the symptoms associated with the trauma or condition.

     What other physical agent modalities could be utilized to treat this injury or condition? Why? How?

Further Discussion Questions

- What is the mechanism of heat transfer in this case?

- What is the effective depth of penetration of the heat using paraffin bath?

- If there had been a significant layer of adipose below the skin, would the physical agent modality selection be the same?

- What are the physiological effects of heat?

- What are the advantages and disadvantages of using paraffin bath for this patient?

- What alternative methods would have achieved the same effect?

Thermotherapy - Infrared Lamp

DESCRIPTION:

Infrared lamps provide superficial (one millimeter or less) heating. Because of the extremely limited penetration, they are not capable of elevating connective tissue temperatures to a therapeutic level. Therefore, their primary effect is one of mild analgesia, and their use is very limited.

PHYSIOLOGICAL EFFECTS:

• Cutaneous vasodilation
• Decreased pain perception

THERAPEUTIC EFFECTS:

• Decreased pain

INDICATIONS:

The principal indication for infrared lamp heating is localized pain. Elevation of skin temperature may decrease the perception of pain for a short period of time.

CONTRAINDICATIONS:

• Lack of normal temperature sensibility
• Peripheral vascular disease with compromised circulation
• Over tumors

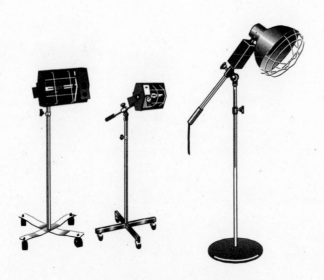

INFRARED LAMP

PROCEDURE	Evaluation #		
	1	2	3
1. Check supplies			
a. Obtain sheet or towels for draping, timer, signaling device.			
b. Check lamp for frayed power cords, integrity of lamp and shields, etc.			
2. Question patient			
a. Verify identity of patient (if not already verified).			
b. Verify the absence of contraindications.			
c. Ask about previous thermotherapy treatments, check treatment notes.			
3. Position patient			
a. Place patient in a well-supported, comfortable position.			
b. Expose body part to be treated, have patient remove all jewelry from the area.			
c. Drape patient to preserve patient's modesty, protect clothing, but allow access to body part.			
4. Inspect body part to be treated			
a. Check light touch perception.			
b. Check circulatory status (pulses, capillary refill).			
c. Verify that there are no open wounds or rashes.			
d. Assess function of body part (e.g., ROM, irritability).			

Checklist continues

PROCEDURE	Evaluation #		
	1	2	3
5. Apply infrared light			
a. Position lamp such that the bulb is parallel to the body part being treated (such that the energy will strike the body at a 90° angle), and is 45 to 60 centimeters away from the patient. Measure and record the distance from the lamp to the closest part of the body being treated.			
b. Inform the patient that they should feel only a mild warmth; if it is hot, they should inform you. Start the lamp.			
c. Set a timer for the appropriate treatment time and give the patient a signaling device. Make sure the patient understands how to use the signaling device.			
d. Check the patient's response after the first five minutes by asking the patient how it feels as well as visually checking the area being treated. Recheck visually and verbally about every 5 minutes.			

Checklist continues

PROCEDURE	Evaluation #		
	1	2	3
6. Complete the treatment			
a. When the treatment time is over, move the lamp away from the patient; dry the area with a towel. Turn the intensity control to zero.			
b. Remove material used for draping, assist the patient in dressing as needed.			
c. Have the patient perform appropriate therapeutic exercise as indicated.			
d. Clean the treatment area and equipment according to normal protocol.			
7. Assess treatment efficacy			
a. Ask the patient how the treated area feels.			
b. Visually inspect the treated area for any adverse reactions.			
c. Perform functional tests as indicated.			

CRYOTHERAPY - Ice Massage

DESCRIPTION:

Ice massage is performed by rubbing a small area of the body with a block of ice until superficial anesthesia is achieved. The block of ice is produced by filling and then freezing a cup of water at a temperature of no colder than - 5° C. Styrofoam cups are often recommended, but the chunks of styrofoam that are removed from the cup during the treatment tend to be messy. Freezing water in empty juice cans with a tongue depressor for a handle are sometimes used, but the tongue depressor may abrade the skin during the treatment. The ideal cup is a waxed paper cup; the wax provides some insulation to keep your hand warm, and half the cup can be torn away in a single piece. The bottom of the cup should be removed, not the top. This permits the cup to act as a funnel, and keeps the ice from slipping out of the cup.

PHYSIOLOGICAL EFFECTS:

- Vasoconstriction
- Anesthesia
- Decreased local metabolism
- Decreased connective tissue elasticity

THERAPEUTIC EFFECTS:

- Decreased or prevented swelling
- Decreased pain
- Decreased inflammation
- Minimized secondary tissue damage

INDICATIONS:

The primary indication for ice massage is pain of musculoskeletal origin that is preventing the effective use of therapeutic exercise. For example, an individual with restricted ankle motion that is prevented from applying sufficient force to produce remodeling of the connective tissue due to pain. Ice massage will decrease the pain enough to permit an effective stretch. However, care must be taken to avoid stressing the connective tissue too much; the anesthesia provided by the ice may allow an overly aggressive individual to produce a sprain or strain.

Ice massage is also useful to help prevent an increase in inflammation and swelling of a joint following a therapeutic exercise session. It is probably no more effective than an ice pack, but often provides a more profound anesthesia.

CONTRAINDICATIONS:

- Lack of normal temperature sensibility
- Cold hypersensitivity (urticaria or hemoglobinuria)
- Vasospastic disorders (e.g., Raynaud's disease)
- Coronary artery disease
- Hypertension

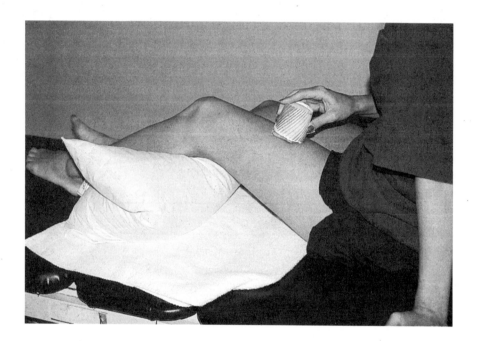

ICE MASSAGE

PROCEDURE	Evaluation #		
	1	2	3
1. Check supplies			
a. Obtain towel to absorb water as it melts, ice cube, sheet or towels for draping.			
b. Check freezer for appropriate temperature.			
2. Question patient			
a. Verify identity of patient (if not already verified).			
b. Verify the absence of contraindications.			
c. Ask about previous cryotherapy treatments, check treatment notes.			
3. Position patient			
a. Place patient in a well-supported, comfortable position.			
b. Expose body part to be treated.			
c. Drape patient to preserve patient's modesty, protect clothing, but allow access to body part.			
4. Inspect body part to be treated			
a. Check light touch perception.			
b. Check circulatory status (pulses, capillary refill).			
c. Verify that there are no open wounds or rashes.			
d. Assess function of body part (e.g., ROM, irritability).			

Checklist continues

PROCEDURE	Evaluation #		
	1	2	3
5. Apply ice massage			
a. Expose block of ice.			
b. Rub ice on hand to smooth rough edges.			
c. Warn the patient that you are going to put your cold hand on the body part to be treated, then do so.			
d. Remove your hand after two or three seconds, and warn the patient that you are going to put the ice on the body part to be treated, then do so.			
e. Begin rubbing the ice block in a circular motion on the body part being treated. Do not put additional pressure on the ice. Move the ice at about five to seven centimeters per second. Do not let melted water run onto areas of the body that are not being treated.			
f. Check the patient's response verbally about every two minutes. Perform a visual check of the area continuously during the treatment. If wheals or welts appear, or if the skin color changes to absolute white within the first four minutes of treatment, stop the treatment. Remind the patient to tell you when the area is numb.			

Checklist continues

PROCEDURE	Evaluation #		
	1	2	3
6. Complete the treatment			
a. When the patient tells you the area is numb, remove the ice and dry the area. Perform a test for light touch sensation to verify anesthesia.			
b. Remove material used for draping, assist the patient in dressing as needed. Place the unused ice in a sink, and the cup in the trash.			
c. Have the patient perform appropriate therapeutic exercise as indicated.			
d. Clean the treatment area and equipment according to normal protocol.			
7. Assess treatment efficacy			
a. Ask the patient how the treated area feels.			
b. Visually inspect the treated area for any adverse reactions (e.g., wheals, welts).			
c. Perform functional tests as indicated.			

Case Study: CRYOTHERAPY - ICE MASSAGE

Background: A 27-year-old novice runner reported to your clinic with a history of rapidly increasing his training mileage to prepare for an upcoming marathon. He admitted that his shoes were pretty worn out, and that he needed to get a new pair. His primary complaint was lateral knee pain, worse at the beginning of a run. He localized the pain just proximal to the lateral joint line. Mild crepitus was palpable during flexion and extension motions. Both the Noble and Ober tests were positive.

Impression: Acute iliotibial band tendinitis.

Treatment Plan: A cup of ice was used to apply ice massage to the lateral aspect of the knee until the patient experienced numbness. The duration of the treatment was approximately 8 minutes. Immediately following the ice massage the patient was instructed to perform static ITB stretching exercises. The patient was advised to obtain new shoes with proper motion control and reduce his training to a minimum level every other day, and to continue with the ice massage and stretching at least 3 times per day.

Response: The patient experienced immediate, transient relief of his pain. He obtained new shoes, and reduced his training mileage and training frequency to every other day. At the 2-week follow-up, the patient was nearly asymptomatic, and was cleared to gradually increase his training regimen.

Discussion Questions for Case Study

- What tissues were injured/affected?
- What symptoms were present?
- What phase of the injury-healing continuum did the patient present for care in?
- What are the physical agent modality's biophysical effects? (direct/indirect/depth/tissue affinity)
- What are the physical agent modality's indications/contraindications?
- What are the parameters of the physical agent modality's application/dosage/duration/ frequency in this case study?

The rehabilitation professional employs physical agent modalities to create an optimum environment for tissue healing while minimizing the symptoms associated with the trauma or condition.

What other physical agent modalities could be utilized to treat this injury or condition? Why? How?

Further Discussion Questions

- What other physical agent modalities could be used to treat this injury or condition? Why? How?

- Was the choice of ice massage optimal for this patient's suspected injury?

- What other things would you counsel this patient to do while undergoing treatment?

- What other techniques could have been used to provide pain management for this patient?

- What are the physiologic mechanisms for the pain relief?

- What effect might the ice massage have on the properties of the tissue being stretched?

Cryotherapy - Ice Pack

DESCRIPTION:

An ice pack uses crushed ice at a temperature of 0 to - 5° C. The ice may be placed in a plastic bag and wrapped in a wet towel, or may be placed directly in a wet towel. The use of a plastic bag will minimize the potential mess from water dripping, but may also decrease the conduction of thermal energy from the patient. A major advantage of an ice pack over a cold pack is that the ice pack can be almost any size and shape; therefore, an ice pack is useful for treating any body part.

PHYSIOLOGICAL EFFECTS:

- Vasoconstriction
- Superficial anesthesia
- Decreased local metabolism
- Decreased connective tissue elasticity

THERAPEUTIC EFFECTS:

- Decreased or reduced swelling
- Decreased pain
- Decreased inflammation
- Decreased secondary tissue damage

INDICATIONS:

The primary indication for the use of an ice pack is in the acute phase of a soft tissue injury. The cooling of the injured area will help prevent the development of swelling, and may assist in the resolution of swelling by altering the Starling-Landis forces at the capillary bed.

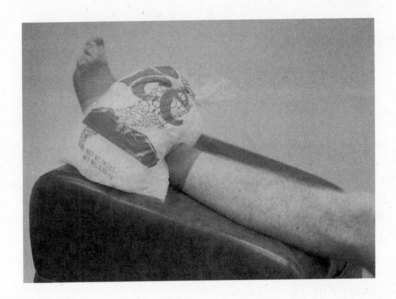

An ice pack is also useful to minimize or prevent increased inflammation or pain following a session of therapeutic exercise. The depth of anesthesia achieved with an ice pack is generally considerably less than with an ice massage.

CONTRAINDICATIONS:
- Lack of normal temperature sensibility
- Cold hypersensitivity (urticaria or hemoglobinuria)
- Vasospastic disorders (e.g., Raynaud's disease)
- Coronary Artery Disease
- Hypertension

ICE PACK

PROCEDURE	Evaluation #		
	1	2	3
1. Check supplies			
a. Obtain wet towel to wrap ice in, an appropriate amount of crushed ice, sheet or towels for draping.			
b. Check freezer for appropriate temperature.			
2. Question patient			
a. Verify identity of patient (if not already verified).			
b. Verify the absence of contraindications.			
c. Ask about previous cryotherapy treatments, check treatment notes.			
3. Position patient			
a. Place patient in a well-supported, comfortable position.			
b. Expose body part to be treated.			
c. Drape patient to preserve patient's modesty, protect clothing, but allow access to body part.			
4. Inspect body part to be treated			
a. Check light touch perception.			
b. Check circulatory status (pulses, capillary refill).			
c. Verify that there are no open wounds or rashes.			
d. Assess function of body part (e.g., ROM, irritability).			

Checklist continues

PROCEDURE	Evaluation #		
	1	2	3
5. Apply ice pack			
a. Warn the patient that you are going to put the ice pack on the body part to be treated, then do so. Make sure the draping will catch any water that melts from the ice pack.			
b. Set a timer for the appropriate treatment time (generally about 20 minutes), and give the patient a signaling device. Make sure the patient understands how to use the signaling device.			
c. Check the patient's response verbally after the first two minutes, then about every 5 minutes. Perform a visual check of the area if the patient reports any unusual sensation. If wheals or welts appear, or if the skin color changes to absolute white within the first four minutes of treatment, stop the treatment.			

Checklist continues

PROCEDURE	Evaluation #		
	1	2	3
6. Complete the treatment			
a. When the treatment time is over, remove the ice pack and dry the area with a towel.			
b. Remove material used for draping, assist the patient in dressing as needed.			
c. Dispose of the used ice in a sink.			
d. Have the patient perform appropriate therapeutic exercise or apply tape or compression wrap as indicated.			
e. Clean the treatment area and equipment according to normal protocol.			
7. Assess treatment efficacy			
a. Ask the patient how the treated area feels.			
b. Visually inspect the treated area for any adverse reactions (e.g., wheals, welts).			
c. Perform functional tests as indicated.			

Cryotherapy - Gel Cold Pack

DESCRIPTION:

Commercially available cold packs are usually a vinyl cover filled with a gel that does not solidify at low temperatures. Cooling units designed specifically for the cold packs are available, but they may be kept in a household type freezer. The temperature of the freezer should be 0 to - 5° C. Packs are available in various sizes, including one designed to encircle the cervical region. The packs are generally wrapped in a wet towel to increase the thermal conductivity from the patient.

PHYSIOLOGICAL EFFECTS:

- Vasoconstriction
- Superficial anesthesia
- Decreased local metabolism
- Decreased connective tissue elasticity

THERAPEUTIC EFFECTS:

- Decreased or reduced swelling
- Decreased pain
- Decreased inflammation
- Decreased secondary tissue damage

INDICATIONS:

The primary indication for the use of a cold pack is in the acute phase of a soft tissue injury. The cooling of the injured area will help prevent the development of swelling, and may assist in the resolution of swelling by altering the Starling-Landis forces at the capillary bed.

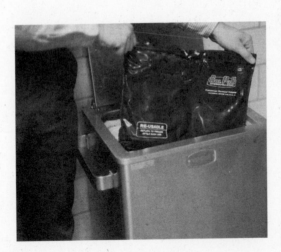
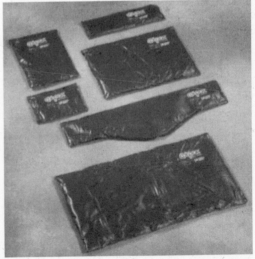

A cold pack is also useful to minimize or prevent increased inflammation or pain following a session of therapeutic exercise. The depth of anesthesia achieved with a cold pack is generally considerably less than with an ice massage.

CONTRAINDICATIONS:

- Lack of normal temperature sensibility
- Cold hypersensitivity (urticaria or hemoglobinuria)
- Vasospastic disorders (e.g., Raynaud's disease)
- Coronary Artery Disease
- Hypertension

GEL COLD PACK

PROCEDURE	Evaluation #		
	1	2	3
1. Check supplies			
a. Obtain wet towel to wrap cold pack in, cold pack, sheet or towels for draping.			
b. Check freezer for appropriate temperature.			
2. Question patient			
a. Verify identity of patient (if not already verified).			
b. Verify the absence of contraindications.			
c. Ask about previous cryotherapy treatments and check treatment notes.			
3. Position patient			
a. Place patient in a well-supported, comfortable position.			
b. Expose body part to be treated.			
c. Drape patient to preserve patient's modesty, protect clothing, but allow access to body part.			
4. Inspect body part to be treated			
a. Check light touch perception.			
b. Check circulatory status (pulses, capillary refill).			
c. Verify that there are no open wounds or rashes.			
d. Assess function of body part (e.g., ROM, irritability).			

Checklist continues

PROCEDURE	Evaluation #		
	1	2	3
5. Apply cold pack			
a. Wrap cold pack in wet towel.			
b. Warn the patient that you are going to put the cold pack on the body part to be treated, then do so.			
c. Set a timer for the appropriate treatment time (generally about 15-20 minutes), and give the patient a signaling device. Make sure the patient understands how to use the signaling device.			
d. Check the patient's response verbally after the first two minutes, then about every 5 minutes. Perform a visual check of the area if the patient reports any unusual sensation. If wheals or welts appear, or if the skin color changes to absolute white within the first four minutes of treatment, stop the treatment.			

Checklist continues

PROCEDURE	Evaluation #		
	1	2	3
6. Complete the treatment			
a. When the treatment time is over, remove the cold pack and dry the area with a towel.			
b. Remove material used for draping, assist the patient in dressing as needed.			
c. Have the patient perform appropriate therapeutic exercise or apply tape or compression wrap as indicated.			
d. Clean the treatment area and equipment according to normal protocol.			
7. Assess treatment efficacy			
a. Ask the patient how the treated area feels.			
b. Visually inspect the treated area for any adverse reactions (e.g., wheals, welts).			
c. Perform functional tests as indicated.			

Case Study: INFRARED PHYSICAL AGENTS

CRYOTHERAPY – ICE MASSAGE, ICE PACK, COLD PACK

Background: A 35-year-old man sustained a Colles fracture of the right wrist during a fall 13 weeks ago. He was treated with a closed reduction and casted for 12 weeks; the cast was removed one week ago. The fracture is well healed with good position. In addition to active and passive exercise, you begin joint mobilization on an every-other-day schedule. In spite of the fact that the tissues are strong enough to tolerate grade II and III mobilization, the patient experiences so much pain that you are limited to grade I mobilization. To increase the patient's tolerance for mobilization, you decide to perform cryotherapy prior to mobilization.

Impression: Limitation of motion and pain secondary to fracture and immobilization.

Treatment Plan: Cryotherapy was applied to the anterior and posterior aspects of the wrist until the patient experienced mild numbness. The duration of the treatment was sufficient to produce the noted analgesia. Immediately following the cryotherapy, joint mobilization techniques were used to increase the range of motion of the wrist.

Response: The patient's tolerance for more aggressive mobilization was increased for approximately 5 minutes following the cryotherapy. As the accessory motions were restored, the active range of motion also improved. After 6 sessions, joint mobilization was discontinued, and the patient continued with active and passive range of motion exercise, and strengthening exercise was added to the program. Ten weeks after removal of the cast, the patient's range of motion in all planes was approximately 90% of normal, and the patient was discharged to a home program.

Discussion Questions for Case Study

- What tissues were injured/affected?
- What symptoms were present?
- What phase of the injury-healing continuum did the patient present for care in?
- What are the physical agent modality's biophysical effects? (direct/indirect/depth/tissue affinity)
- What are the physical agent modality's indications/contraindications?
- What are the parameters of the physical agent modality's application/dosage/duration/ frequency in this case study?
- Which form of cryotherapy would you think would be most effective in addressing the patient's symptoms which were interfering with restoration of wrist motion? Why?

The rehabilitation professional employs physical agent modalities to create an optimum environment for tissue healing while minimizing the symptoms associated with the trauma or condition.

What other physical agent modalities could be utilized to treat this injury or condition? Why? How?

Further Discussion Questions

- What other techniques could have been used to provide pain management for the joint mobilization?

- What are the physiological mechanisms for the pain relief?

- Why was it necessary to begin the joint mobilization immediately following the cryotherapy?

- What effect might the cryotherapy have on the properties of the tissues being mobilized? Is there another treatment that would have the opposite effect?

Cryotherapy - Vapocoolant Spray

DESCRIPTION:

Vapocoolant sprays, such as Fluori-Methane and ethyl chloride, are liquids that are sprayed on the skin. Thermal energy from the body is absorbed by the liquids, which have low boiling points; therefore, the liquid almost immediately evaporates. As it evaporates, thermal energy is removed from the body, resulting in a superficial cooling.

Fluori-Methane, a mixture of 85% trichloromonofluoromethane and 15% dichlorodifluoromethane, is not flammable and is nontoxic. Ethyl chloride is flammable, and is therefore not recommended for use.

PHYSIOLOGICAL EFFECTS:

- Superficial anesthesia

THERAPEUTIC EFFECTS:

- Inhibition of painful trigger points
- Decrease in pain with stretching musculotendinous tissue

INDICATIONS:

Vapocoolant sprays are used mostly for the treatment of trigger points and for stretching of tight musculotendinous tissue. Trigger points are a poorly understood phenomenon, but many pain syndromes are ascribed to active trigger points. Two relatively common treatments for trigger points are deep friction massage (similar to vigorous acupressure) and stretching of the muscle the trigger point is located within. Because direct pressure on and stretching of the trigger points is painful, the area can be sprayed with a vapocoolant to decrease the pain during the treatment.

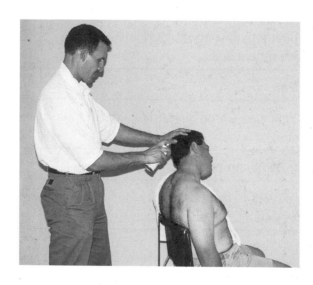

In a similar manner, if a musculotendinous strain has resulted in a loss of range of motion, spraying the skin over the injured muscle may decrease the pain perception while the therapist stretches the body part. Care must be taken to not overstretch the tissue and produce further injury.

CONTRAINDICATIONS:

- Lack of normal temperature sensibility
- Cold hypersensitivity (urticaria or hemoglobinuria)
- Vasospastic disorders (e.g., Raynaud's disease)

VAPOCOOLANT SPRAY

PROCEDURE	Evaluation #		
	1	2	3
1. Check supplies			
a. Obtain vapocoolant.			
b. Obtain toweling or other draping materials needed.			
2. Question patient			
a. Verify identity of patient (if not already verified).			
b. Verify the absence of contraindications.			
c. Ask about previous cryotherapy treatments, check treatment notes.			
3. Position patient			
a. Place patient in a well-supported, comfortable position.			
b. Expose body part to be treated.			
c. Drape patient to preserve patient's modesty, protect clothing, but allow access to body part.			

Checklist continues

PROCEDURE	Evaluation #		
	1	2	3
4. Inspect body part to be treated			
a. Check light touch perception.			
b. Check circulatory status (pulses, capillary refill).			
c. Verify that there are no open wounds or rashes.			
d. Assess function of body part (e.g., ROM, irritability).			
5. Apply vapocoolant			
a. Position body part such that the area to be treated is on a stretch.			
b. Protect the patient's eyes, and insure the patient does not inhale fumes.			
c. Holding the vapocoolant upside down, with the nozzle at about a 30° angle from the perpendicular with the skin, and about 45 cm from the skin, spray the skin from distal to proximal.			
d. Spray in one direction only 3 to 4 times, then apply direct pressure or increased stretch as indicated and tolerated by the patient. Repeat the procedure as needed after the skin has rewarmed.			
e. Check the patient's response frequently during the treatment.			

Checklist continues

PROCEDURE	Evaluation #		
	1	2	3
6. Complete treatment			
a. Upon attainment of the desired therapeutic effect (or up to 4 repetitions of spray and stretch or pressure, or to patient tolerance), inspect the treated body part for adverse reactions.			
b. Remove draping materials, assist the patient in dressing as needed.			
c. If further therapeutic exercise is indicated, instruct the patient to perform it.			
d. Clean the treatment area and equipment according to normal protocol.			
7. Assess treatment efficacy			
a. Ask the patient how the treated area feels.			
b. Visually inspect the treated area for any adverse reactions (e.g., wheals, welts).			
c. Perform functional tests as indicated.			

HYDROTHERAPY - Warm Whirlpool

DESCRIPTION:

A whirlpool is a tank filled with water of a particular temperature, depending on the desired therapeutic effect. The tank also contains a turbine or pump that creates convection currents in the water. Although water that is any temperature above the temperature of the body surface could be considered "warm", generally water at 35 - 43° C is used. If the entire body is to be immersed, temperatures above 38° C should not be used to avoid interference with thermoregulation. The use of the turbine avoids the development of a layer of cooler water adjacent to the body part, thus producing more uniform warming. Because of the dependent position of the body part in the whirlpool and the increased temperature of the body part, a warm whirlpool may increase soft tissue swelling; even in non-injured limbs, there may be a considerable increase in interstitial fluid following a warm whirlpool.

Because the turbine is powered by electricity, it is generally prudent to not let the patient touch any part of the turbine. Also, patients should not be left in the whirlpool unattended; this is true whether the entire body or only a limb is immersed.

PHYSIOLOGICAL EFFECTS:

- Vasodilation
- Decreased pain perception
- Increased local metabolism
- Increased connective tissue plasticity
- Decreased isometric strength (transient)

THERAPEUTIC EFFECTS:

- Decreased pain
- Increased soft tissue extensibility
- Sedative

INDICATIONS:

The principal indication for a warm whirlpool is to provide therapeutic warming of a larger area of the body than can be achieved readily with a hot pack. The effective depth of therapeutic heating is the same at approximately one cm. In addition, the patient can perform active exercise during the application, or the therapist can perform joint mobilization on the injured limb while immersed in the water. Some therapists use whirlpool for cleaning a limb after removal of a cast; equally effective and at less cost is a shower.

The primary therapeutic effect of superficial heating is to increase the ability of the collagen to remodel. Therefore, heating the tissue is beneficial following a period of reduced mobility if the soft tissue has shortened. In addition, the tissue viscosity is reduced, resulting in a greater ease of motion through the available range of motion.

CONTRAINDICATIONS:

- Lack of normal temperature sensibility
- Peripheral vascular disease with compromised circulation
- Over tumors
- Coronary artery disease

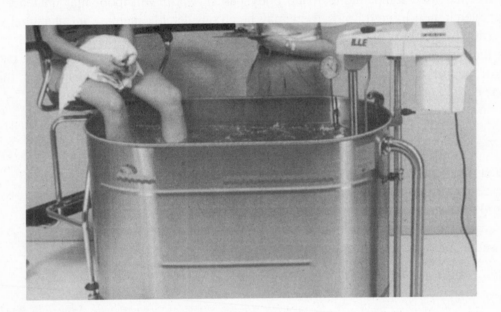

WARM WHIRLPOOL

PROCEDURE	Evaluation #		
	1	2	3
1. Check supplies and equipment			
a. Obtain towels for padding the edge of the whirlpool tank, as well as for drying the treated part.			
b. Check temperature of tank before applying treatment.			
c. Position chair of correct height next to whirlpool.			
2. Question patient			
a. Verify identity of patient (if not already verified).			
b. Verify the absence of contraindications.			
c. Ask about previous thermotherapy or whirlpool treatments, check treatment notes.			
3. Position patient			
a. Have patient sit on chair with body part out of water.			
b. Expose body part to be treated.			
c. Drape patient to preserve patient's modesty, protect clothing, but allow access to body part.			
4. Inspect body part to be treated			
a. Check light touch perception.			
b. Check circulatory status (pulses, capillary refill).			
c. Verify that there are no open wounds or rashes.			
d. Assess function of body part (e.g., ROM, irritability).			

Checklist continues

PROCEDURE	Evaluation #		
	1	2	3
5. Administer warm whirlpool			
a. Pad edge of tank with toweling, ask patient to tell you if the water is too hot, then place body part in water.			
b. Instruct patient to keep away from all parts of the turbine.			
c. Turn on the turbine, adjust the aeration, agitation, and direction of the water being pumped.			
d. Check the patient's response verbally and visually about every two minutes. Remind the patient to tell you if the area starts hurting or if sensation is lost.			
6. Complete the treatment			
a. Turn off the turbine at the completion of the treatment time.			
b. Remove the body part from the water and dry it off.			
c. Assist the patient in dressing as needed, and instruct in therapeutic exercise as indicated.			
d. Clean the treatment area and equipment according to normal protocol.			
7. Assess treatment efficacy			
a. Ask the patient how the treated area feels.			
b. Visually inspect the treated area for any adverse reactions (e.g., wheals, welts).			
c. Perform functional tests as indicated.			

Case Study: HYDROTHERAPY - WARM WHIRLPOOL

Background: An 82-year-old man who regularly participated in mountain hiking underwent bilateral total knee arthroplasty six weeks ago. He was treated in the hospital post-operatively with strengthening and range of motion exercise, and gait and ADL training. His range of motion at hospital discharge was 5/90 bilaterally, and he was independent in ambulation with a walker. Arrangements for home health visits were completed prior to discharge; however, due to an administrative error, no visits were made. Two days ago, the patient returned to the orthopaedic surgeon, who noted that the patient had bilateral flexion contractures, limiting his knee motion to 45/70 bilaterally. The patient was referred to you for aggressive range of motion and strengthening exercise. He is ambulating independently with a walker, though he walks with both hips and knees flexed. His incisions are completely healed, and there is no joint effusion. He has no significant cardiovascular or pulmonary disorders.

Impression: Severe post-operative limitation of motion of both knees.

Treatment Plan: Active, Active-Assistive, and Passive (stretching) Range of Motion in a "lowboy" whirlpool, with water temperature at 38 degrees C for 30 minutes, three days per week. For the initial 10 minutes, the patient was instructed to actively flex and extend the knees, using the buoyancy of the water to help extend the knees. The next 10 minutes consisted of gentle overpressure at the end of the available range of motion (active-assistive), and the final 10 minutes consisted of more forceful static stretching into both flexion and extension. In addition, generalized and specific strengthening exercises were performed, as well as additional gait training.

Response: There was a gradual increase in knee range of motion over the course of eight weeks; after 24 visits, the patient was discharged to a home program. His knee range of motion was 0/110 bilaterally, and he was ambulating independently with a single cane.

Discussion Questions for Case Study

- What tissues were injured/affected?
- What symptoms were present?
- What phase of the injury-healing continuum did the patient present for care in?
- What are the physical agent modality's biophysical effects? (direct/indirect/depth/tissue affinity)
- What are the physical agent modality's indications/contraindications?
- What are the parameters of the physical agent modality's application/dosage/duration/ frequency in this case study?
- Which form of cryotherapy would you think would be most effective in addressing the patient's symptoms which were interfering with restoration of wrist motion? Why?

The rehabilitation professional employs physical agent modalities to create an optimum environment for tissue healing while minimizing the symptoms associated with the trauma or condition.

What other physical agent modalities could be utilized to treat this injury or condition? Why? How?

Further Discussion Questions

- If the patient had significant effusion of the knee joints, would the warm whirlpool have been the optimal physical agent of choice? Why or why not?

- What would the effect of the exposure to warm water have been on the physiologic mechanisms of the effusion?

- If the patient's incisions were not fully healed, would his treatment have been altered? Why or why not?

- What unique features of the whirlpool need to be considered in the case of open wounds?

- Why was a "lowboy" chosen? What advantages and disadvantages are there to a "lowboy" versus and "large extremity" whirlpool for this patient?

- If the patient had co-existing cardiovascular pathology (e.g., heart failure, peripheral vascular disease), would the ideal treatment have been different? Why or why not?

Hydrotherapy - Cold Whirlpool

DESCRIPTION:

A whirlpool is a tank filled with water of a particular temperature, depending on the desired therapeutic effect. The tank also contains a turbine or pump that creates convection currents in the water. Although water that is any temperature below the temperature of the body surface could be considered "cold", generally water at 10 - 16° C is used. Because water from the tap is rarely this cold, ice must be added to the tank. Crushed ice results in the most rapid cooling of the water, and *all ice must be melted before the turbine is turned on.* Using the turbine insures that a layer of warm water does not develop adjacent to the skin, thus providing a more effective cooling of the tissues. Because the limb is in a dependent position, any effect of the cooling on decreasing soft tissue swelling may be negated; using a compression bandage during the treatment may help in reducing the effects of dependency. As with a warm whirlpool, the patient should not be left unattended, and should be warned against touching any part of the turbine.

PHYSIOLOGICAL EFFECTS:

- Vasoconstriction
- Superficial anesthesia
- Decreased local metabolism
- Decreased connective tissue elasticity

THERAPEUTIC EFFECTS:

- Decreased or prevented swelling
- Decreased pain
- Decreased inflammation
- Decreased secondary tissue damage

INDICATIONS:

The principal indication for a cold whirlpool is to provide therapeutic cooling of a larger area of the body than can be achieved readily with an ice or cold pack. Also, irregular shaped areas of the body can be treated with total contact. In addition, the patient can perform active exercise during the application, or the therapist can perform joint mobilization on the injured limb while immersed in the water.

In addition, use of a cold whirlpool may minimize inflammation and swelling following a therapeutic exercise session. The advantage of a cold whirlpool over an ice or cold pack is the greater area that can be treated; a disadvantage is the possibility of increased swelling when the limb is in a dependent position.

CONTRAINDICATIONS:

- Lack of normal temperature sensibility
- Cold hypersensitivity (urticaria or hemoglobinuria)
- Vasospastic disorders (e.g., Raynaud's disease)
- Coronary artery disease
- Hypertension

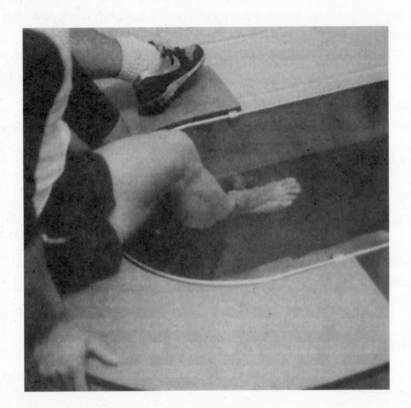

COLD WHIRLPOOL

PROCEDURE		Evaluation #		
		1	2	3
1. Check supplies and equipment				
	a. Obtain towels for padding the edge of the whirlpool tank, as well as for drying the treated part.			
	b. Check temperature of tank, ensure all ice is melted before applying treatment.			
	c. Position chair of correct height next to whirlpool.			
2. Question patient				
	a. Verify identity of patient (if not already verified).			
	b. Verify the absence of contraindications.			
	c. Ask about previous cryotherapy or whirlpool treatments, check treatment notes.			
3. Position patient				
	a. Have patient sit on chair with body part out of water.			
	b. Expose body part to be treated.			
	c. Drape patient to preserve patient's modesty, protect clothing, but allow access to body part.			
4. Inspect body part to be treated				
	a. Check light touch perception.			
	b. Check circulatory status (pulses, capillary refill).			
	c. Verify that there are no open wounds or rashes.			
	d. Assess function of body part (e.g., ROM, irritability).			

Checklist continues

PROCEDURE	Evaluation #		
	1	2	3
5. Administer cold whirlpool			
a. Pad edge of tank with toweling, warn patient that the water is cold, then place body part in water.			
b. Instruct patient to keep away from all parts of the turbine.			
c. Turn on the turbine, adjust the aeration, agitation, and direction of the water being pumped.			
d. Check the patient's response verbally and visually about every two minutes. Remind the patient to tell you if the area starts hurting or if sensation is lost.			
6. Complete the treatment			
a. Turn off the turbine at the completion of the treatment time.			
b. Remove the body part from the water and dry it off.			
c. Assist the patient in dressing as needed, and instruct in therapeutic exercise as indicated.			
d. Clean the treatment area and equipment according to normal protocol.			
7. Assess treatment efficacy			
a. Ask the patient how the treated area feels.			
b. Visually inspect the treated area for any adverse reactions (e.g., wheals, welts).			
c. Perform functional tests as indicated.			

Case Study: HYDROTHERAPY - COLD WHIRLPOOL

Background: A 32-year-old woman fell onto her outstretched left hand 12 weeks ago while playing tennis, and sustained a comminuted fracture of the distal radius as well as a non-comminuted fracture of the scaphoid. She was treated with a closed reduction and external fixation (fiberglass cast) for 8 weeks, then a splint for 4 weeks. She has been referred for rehabilitation, to include mobilization, strengthening, and range-of-motion exercise. The radius demonstrates radiographic healing, and there is no evidence of aseptic necrosis. Her distal forearm, wrist, hand, and fingers remain markedly swollen, and she is experiencing significant pain at rest. She is unable to tolerate more than mild pressure on the wrist, making joint mobilization extremely difficult, and has severe pain with attempted active range of motion.

Impression: Posttraumatic pain and swelling, postimmobilization pain and loss of motion.

Treatment Plan: A small extremity hydrotherapy tank was filled with ice and water to achieve a water temperature of 17° C (63° F). The patient's left upper member was immersed in the water up to the level of the mid-forearm, and the turbine was used to direct water onto the wrist and hand. For the initial 5 minutes, the patient was instructed to gently move the wrist and hand actively. For the next 5 minutes, passive range of motion was conducted by the therapist; 5 minutes of joint mobilization followed the passive range of motion. The total treatment time in the cold whirlpool was 15 minutes. She was instructed in a home exercise program to gain motion and strength.

Response: The patient was treated with the cold whirlpool 3 days per week for 3 weeks, at which time the swelling had subsided to a minimal amount. Her range of motion was approximately 50 percent that of the right wrist and hand. The cold whirlpool was discontinued after 9 sessions, and other physical agents were used to facilitate a return to function. After an additional 12 sessions, the patient was discharged to a home program, with her left wrist and hand motion and strength approximately 80 percent of the right wrist and hand. She had returned to low-level activity on the tennis court, using a custom-fitted semi-rigid splint on the wrist for protection.

Discussion Questions for Case Study

- What tissues were injured/affected?
- What symptoms were present?
- What phase of the injury-healing continuum did the patient present for care in?
- What are the physical agent modality's biophysical effects? (direct/indirect/depth/tissue affinity)
- What are the physical agent modality's indications/contraindications?
- What are the parameters of the physical agent modality's application/dosage/duration/ frequency in this case study?
- Which form of cryotherapy would you think would be most effective in addressing the patient's symptoms which were interfering with restoration of wrist motion? Why?

The rehabilitation professional employs physical agent modalities to create an optimum environment for tissue healing while minimizing the symptoms associated with the trauma or condition.

What other physical agent modalities could be utilized to treat this injury or condition? Why? How?

Further Discussion Questions

- What is aseptic necrosis? Are particular areas more vulnerable? What areas? What is the mechanism of the disorder?

- What does the abbreviation "FOOSH" stand for? What types of injuries would you anticipate in a patient who had experiences a "FOOSH"?

- If the cold whirlpool was helpful in achieving the therapeutic goals, why was the cold whirlpool discontinued after 9 sessions?

- Why was a cold whirlpool selected for this patient?

- What disadvantages are there in using a whirlpool to assist in the resolution of the soft tissue swelling? Advantages?

- If the patient had coexisting cardiovascular pathology (e.g., heart failure, peripheral vascular disease), would the ideal treatment have been different? Why or why not?

- What effect does the water driven by the turbine have on the ability of the patient to tolerate the aggressive stretching? What is the mechanism for this effect?

Hydrotherapy - Contrast Bath

DESCRIPTION:

A contrast bath involves the alternating immersion of the involved body part in warm water and cold water. Usually, the wrist and hand or foot and ankle are treated, though the entire upper or lower member could be treated using two whirlpool tanks. The duration of immersion in each temperature water is variable, as is the number of times immersed during a single treatment session. A suggested sequence is to start with three minutes in warm, followed by one minute in cold, with the sequence repeated 5 times (e.g., 3W-1C-3W-1C-3W-1C-3W-1C-3W-1C); however, some therapists recommend starting and ending with warm water. The warm water should be 40 - 41° C, and the cold water 10 - 16° C.

PHYSIOLOGICAL EFFECTS:

- Alternating vasodilation and vasoconstriction

THERAPEUTIC EFFECTS:

- Variable effects on swelling
- Decreased pain

INDICATIONS:

Contrast baths are often used in the sub-acute and chronic stages of recovery. Most of the information regarding benefits of contrast baths is anecdotal; there is little research documenting the efficacy of this treatment.

CONTRAINDICATIONS:

- Lack of normal temperature sensibility
- Cold hypersensitivity (urticaria or hemoglobinuria)
- Vasospastic disorders (e.g., Raynaud's disease)

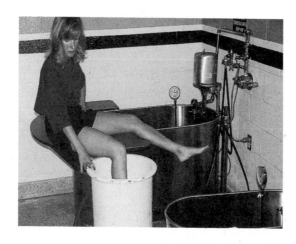

CONTRAST BATH

PROCEDURE	Evaluation #		
	1	2	3
1. Check supplies and equipment			
a. Obtain towels, containers, ice, timer, etc.			
b. Check temperature of water in each container.			
2. Question patient			
a. Verify identity of patient (if not already verified).			
b. Verify the absence of contraindications.			
c. Ask about previous cryotherapy or thermotherapy treatments, check treatment notes.			
3. Position patient			
a. Have patient sit in a comfortable position.			
b. Expose body part to be treated.			
c. Drape patient to preserve patient's modesty, protect clothing, but allow access to body part.			
4. Inspect body part to be treated			
a. Check light touch perception.			
b. Check circulatory status (pulses, capillary refill).			
c. Verify that there are no open wounds or rashes.			
d. Assess function of body part (e.g., ROM, irritability).			

Checklist continues

PROCEDURE	Evaluation #		
	1	2	3
5. Administer contrast bath			
a. Set timer for appropriate interval, help patient immerse body part fully into warm water; start timer.			
b. After the timer goes off, set it for the next interval. Warn patient that the cold water will feel very cold; help patient immerse body part fully into cold water; start timer.			
c. Continue the cycles until the treatment is complete. Usually, the patient can time each immersion themselves.			
d. Check the patient's response verbally and visually about every two minutes. Remind the patient to tell you if the area starts hurting or if sensation is lost.			
6. Complete the treatment			
a. Remove the body part from the water and dry it off.			
b. Assist the patient in dressing as needed, and instruct in therapeutic exercise as indicated.			
c. Clean the treatment area and equipment according to normal protocol.			
7. Assess treatment efficacy			
a. Ask the patient how the treated area feels.			
b. Visually inspect the treated area for any adverse reactions (e.g., wheals, welts).			
c. Perform functional tests as indicated.			

Case Study #1: HYDROTHERAPY - CONTRAST BATH

Background: A 29-year-old man sustained a laceration of the right posterior forearm in a roller-blading accident. There was a partial laceration of the extensor carpi radialis longus, the extensor carpi radialis brevis, and the extensor digitorum (communis), no arterial damage, no motor nerve damage, but a complete transection of the superficial radial nerve. The laceration was sutured primarily, and a splint applied to prevent stress on the repair. The patient is now 12 weeks postinjury, and has full wrist and hand motion, and near-normal strength. However, he has developed extreme sensitivity to any stimulus over the dorsal-radial aspect of the wrist and hand, and experiences severe pain when anything touches the area (including a breeze). The area innervated by the superficial radial nerve is glossy in appearance, and is now hairless (as compared to the left forearm and hand). He has been referred for pain management and desensitization.

Impression: Complex regional pain syndrome (CRPS) type II (also known as causalgia).

Treatment Plan: Two basins large enough to immerse the entire forearm were filled with water, one at 40°C (104°F) and the other at 14°C (57°F). The patient's forearm was immersed in the warm water for 2 minutes, then removed and immersed in the cold water for 1 minute. The sequence was repeated 6 times, for a total treatment duration of 18 minutes. Immediately after the final immersion, the patient was encouraged to brush the painful area with his left hand, and to tap over the mid- and distal-radius, along the course of the superficial radial nerve.

Response: After the initial treatment, the patient noted little improvement, and was unable to tolerate the desensitization. The treatment was repeated the next day, and he was able to tolerate a few seconds of desensitization. He was treated in the clinic daily for a total of 4 sessions, and was then instructed to continue the contrast bath treatment on a home program, with weekly rechecks. He completed twice-daily sessions at home, and noted very gradual increases in the duration of the increased tolerance to touch and tapping, as well as an ability to tolerate more vigorous touch. Two months later, there was no hypersensitivity in the superficial radial nerve distribution, and the skin had returned to a normal appearance.

Case Study #2: HYDROTHERAPY - CONTRAST BATH

Background: A 12-year-old select male soccer player sustained a bimalleolar fracture of his left ankle during an indoor tournament 6 weeks ago. He was treated with an open reduction internal fixation of the fractures with cast immobilization and non-weightbearing for 6 weeks. The cast was removed yesterday with a referral to you to initiate care. He demonstrates only 5 degrees of dorsiflexion and 20 degrees of plantarflexion at the talocrural joint. Inversion and eversion are non existent at this time. The surgical incisions appear to be healing well. The forefoot exhibits a moderate amount of soft tissue edema and a figure 8 measure of the joint indicates that it is 1 and 1/4 inches larger than the uninvolved side which is attributed to joint effusion. To initiate the patient's rehabilitation; facilitate edema and effusion resorption and encourage range of motion, you decide to employ hydrotherapy as an initial treatment.

Impression: Limitation of motion secondary to fracture, surgery and immobilization.

Treatment Plan: Because the target tissues are immediately sub-cutaneous and the foot and ankle are swollen you elect to use contrast bath. Following standard protocol, the patient performed a contrast bath regimen for the left ankle. Immediately after completion of the contrast bath, active and passive range of motion exercise was initiated. Progressive weightbearing was also initiated.

Response: The patient performed contrast bath prior to exercising on a daily basis for 3 weeks. Effusion and edema resolved and ankle AROM measures were within normal limits. Weightbearing status was full and was advanced into a full ankle strengthening and functional rehabilitation regimen.

Discussion Questions for Case Studies

* What tissues were injured/affected?
* What symptoms were present?
* What phase of the injury-healing continuum did the patient present for care in?
* What are the physical agent modality's biophysical effects? (direct/indirect/depth/tissue affinity)
* What are the physical agent modality's indications/contraindications?
* What are the parameters of the physical agent modality's application/dosage/duration/frequency in this case study?
* Which form of cryotherapy would you think would be most effective in addressing the patient's symptoms which were interfering with restoration of wrist motion? Why?

The rehabilitation professional employs physical agent modalities to create an optimum environment for tissue healing while minimizing the symptoms associated with the trauma or condition.

What other physical agent modalities could be utilized to treat this injury or condition? Why? How?

Further Discussion Questions

- What is the mechanism of physiologic action in these cases?

- What is the effective depth of effect of contrast bath?

- If there had been a delay in healing of the skin, would the physical agent modality selection be the same?

- What are the advantages and disadvantages of using contrast baths for these types of patients?

- Would alternative methods such as warm or cold whirlpool have achieved the same effect?

- What is CRPS type II?

- What is the difference between CRPS type I and CRPS type II?

- Is it likely that CRPS could have been prevented in this patient? How?

- If the patient's fingertips had become very pale during the immersion in the cold water, and the patient had complained of severe pain in the fingertips, what would have been your response? What pathology would you suspect?

Hydrotherapy - Fluidotherapy®

DESCRIPTION:

Fluidotherapy® is a device manufactured by Chattanooga Corporation, Chattanooga, Tennessee. Heated air is forced through a container filled with cellulose particles; when heated, the cellulose takes on fluid-like characteristics. The body part to be treated is immersed in the cellulose particles, and the particles are circulated in the container, thus providing elevation of tissue temperature and a mechanical stimulation of the skin. The temperature of the unit is adjustable within a range of about 39 to 48° C.

There are several advantages to using Fluidotherapy® to treat affected hands or feet. The source of heat is constant, so the tissue temperature can be maintained at a therapeutic level for the duration of the treatment. The body part can be exercised either actively or passively by the therapist during the treatment. The mechanical stimulation of the skin with the cellulose particles may provide some analgesic effect, and may help desensitize the injured area.

PHYSIOLOGICAL EFFECTS:

- Vasodilation
- Decreased pain perception
- Increased local metabolism
- Increased connective tissue plasticity
- Decreased isometric strength (transient)

THERAPEUTIC EFFECTS:

- Decreased pain
- Increased soft tissue extensibility

INDICATIONS:

The principal indication for Fluidotherapy® is to provide therapeutic warming of a larger area of the body than can be achieved readily with a hot pack. In addition, the patient can perform active exercise during the application, or the therapist can perform joint mobilization on the injured limb while in the unit.

The primary therapeutic effect of superficial heating is to increase the ability of the collagen to remodel. Therefore, heating the tissue is beneficial following a period of reduced mobility if the soft tissue has shortened. In addition, the tissue viscosity is reduced, resulting in a greater ease of motion through the available range of motion.

CONTRAINDICATIONS:

- Lack of normal temperature sensibility
- Peripheral vascular disease with compromised circulation
- Over tumors
- Coronary artery disease

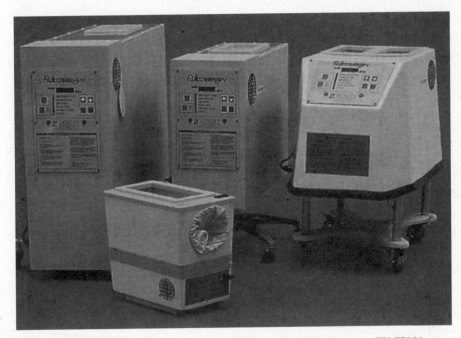

Photo courtesy of Fluidotherapy Corporation, 6113 Aletha Lane, Houston, TX 77081.

FLUIDOTHERAPY®

PROCEDURE	Evaluation #		
	1	2	3
1. Check supplies and equipment			
a. Obtain timer, signaling device, etc.			
b. Check temperature of Fluidotherapy® unit before applying treatment.			
c. Position chair of correct height next to unit.			
2. Question patient			
a. Verify identity of patient (if not already verified).			
b. Verify the absence of contraindications.			
c. Ask about previous thermotherapy treatments, check treatment notes.			
3. Position patient			
a. Have patient remove jewelry from area to be treated and thoroughly wash and dry area.			
b. Have patient sit on chair next to unit.			
c. Expose body part to be treated.			
d. Drape patient to preserve patient's modesty, protect clothing, but allow access to body part.			
4. Inspect body part to be treated			
a. Check light touch perception.			
b. Check circulatory status (pulses, capillary refill).			
c. Verify that there are no open wounds or rashes.			

Checklist continues

PROCEDURE	Evaluation #		
	1	2	3
d. Assess function of body part (e.g., ROM, irritability).			
5. Administer Fluidotherapy®			
a. With the agitation off, open the sleeved portion of the unit.			
b. Instruct patient to insert body part into cellulose particles, reminding them to tell you if the temperature is too hot.			
c. Fasten the sleeve around the body part to prevent the cellulose particles from being blown out of the unit, and start the agitation.			
d. Check the patient's response verbally after about five minutes. Remind the patient to tell you if the heating sensation becomes uncomfortable.			
e. Instruct the patient in any indicated therapeutic exercise to be performed during the treatment.			
6. Complete the treatment			
a. Turn off the agitation at the completion of the treatment time.			
b. Remove the body part from the unit, having the patient brush or shake off as much of the cellulose as possible.			
c. Assist the patient in dressing as needed, and instruct in therapeutic exercise as indicated.			
d. Clean the treatment area and equipment according to normal protocol.			

Checklist continues

PROCEDURE	Evaluation #		
	1	2	3
7. Assess treatment efficacy			
a. Ask the patient how the treated area feels.			
b. Visually inspect the treated area for any adverse reactions (e.g., wheals, welts).			
c. Perform functional tests as indicated.			

Chapter 7: ULTRAVIOLET THERAPY

DESCRIPTION:

Electromagnetic energy in the ultraviolet (UV) wavelength range has several medically accepted uses; however, it is rare for a sports therapist to treat a patient with ultraviolet. In the past, UV was considered a heating physical agent because of the sensation of warmth that is produced. However, the warmth is extremely superficial, and UV is not considered a heating physical agent.

UV energy is absorbed by the epidermis, and to a limited extent the dermis. The primary effect is to produce an increase in the synthesis of vitamins D_2 and D_3, and an increase in melanin content of the epidermis as a protective response.

There is also evidence that UV energy stimulates cells of the reticuloendothelial system in the dermis of the skin. This may enhance the immune response to bacterial infection, thus helping the body overcome the infection.

Prior to initiating a course of treatment with UV, the individual patient's sensitivity to UV must be determined. Because the total energy delivered to the patient is a function of the duration of exposure, the distance from the source to the patient, and the angle of intercept of the UV light with the skin, two of these three variables must remain constant. The easiest one to vary is the time of exposure; therefore, distance and angle should remain constant from the time of determination of appropriate dosage throughout the duration of the treatment. The appropriate beginning dose of UV is the time, distance, and angle that produces a minimal erythemal dose (MED). One MED is the time of exposure that produces an erythemal reaction within eight hours of exposure and that disappears within 24 hours of exposure. This can be determined by exposing an area of skin that is not normally exposed to sunlight (e.g., the anterior surface of the forearm, lower abdomen) to UV for specific durations. The best way to do this is to cover the area with paper or cloth that has six small (approximately one cm diameter) holes cut in it; five of the holes are covered, while the skin exposed by the sixth hole is exposed to the UV for 30 seconds. After 30 seconds, the adjacent hole is uncovered for 30 seconds, then another hole is uncovered every 15 seconds. This results in exposures of 120, 105, 90, 75, 60, and 30 seconds. The areas exposed should be marked so that the patient can report which area turns red within eight hours and resolves within 24 hours.

PHYSIOLOGICAL EFFECTS:

- Vitamin D synthesis enhanced
- Melanin deposition enhanced
- Bacteriocidal

THERAPEUTIC EFFECTS:

- Skeletal deposition of calcium enhanced
- Desquamation of epithelium enhanced
- Infectious organisms may be destroyed

INDICATIONS:

The principal indications for UV radiation are dermatological conditions such as psoriasis and acne. Dietary approaches are generally used to correct Vitamin D deficiencies.

CONTRAINDICATIONS:

- Hypersensitivity to UV radiation

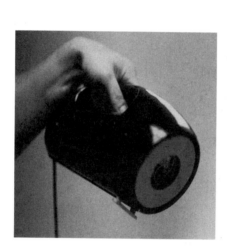
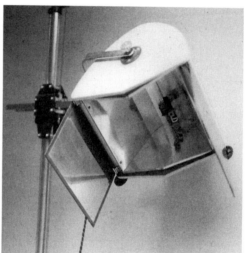
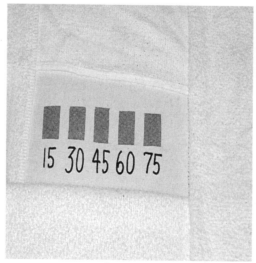

ULTRAVIOLET THERAPY

PROCEDURE	Evaluation #		
	1	2	3
1. Check supplies			
a. Obtain sheet or towels for draping, stopwatch, UV protection goggles for patient and therapist.			
b. Check lamp for frayed power cords, integrity of lamp and shields, etc.			
c. Verify that the intensity control is at zero.			
2. Question patient			
a. Verify identity of patient (if not already verified).			
b. Verify the absence of contraindications.			
c. Ask about previous ultraviolet treatments, check treatment notes.			
3. Position patient			
a. Place patient in a well-supported, comfortable position.			
b. Expose body part to be treated, have patient remove all jewelry from the area.			
c. Drape patient to preserve patient's modesty, protect clothing, but allow access to body part. Insure that only the area you want to expose to UV is exposed; draping is crucial.			
4. Inspect body part to be treated			
a. Check for precancerous skin lesions (e.g., keratoses).			

Checklist continues

PROCEDURE	Evaluation #		
	1	2	3
b. If treating for acne, attempt to quantify the number of lesions; if treating a wound, measure the size of the wound.			
5. Determine Minimal Erythemal Dose (MED) of ultraviolet light on initial treatment day.			
a. Cut 6 one-cm^2 holes of different shaped in a piece of cloth (e.g., stockinette) or stiff paper (e.g., file folder).			
b. Cover an area of the body away from the treatment area that has not been exposed to ultraviolet in the past few weeks (e.g., the abdomen or anterior forearm) with the paper or cloth.			
c. Position lamp such that the bulb is parallel to the body part being treated (such that the energy will strike the body at a 90° angle), and is about 75 centimeters away from the patient.			
d. Inform the patient that they should feel only a mild warmth; if it is hot, they should inform you. Start the lamp.			
e. Expose the first window for 30 seconds, then uncover the second window for an additional 30 seconds; continue exposing remaining windows every 15 seconds. If 6 windows are used, the first window will have been exposed for 120 seconds the last for only 15 seconds.			

Checklist continues

PROCEDURE	Evaluation #		
	1	2	3
g. The MED is the duration of exposure that produces redness within 8 hours and disappears within 24 hours. Inform the patient to inspect the test area over the next 24 hour period, and report the results on the next visit.			
5b. Apply ultraviolet light			
a. Position lamp such that the bulb is parallel to the body part being treated (such that the energy will strike the body at a 90° angle), and is about 75 centimeters away from the patient.			
b. Inform the patient that they should feel only a mild warmth; if it is hot, they should inform you. Start the lamp.			
c. Expose the treatment area for the appropriate time (i.e., one MED for the first treatment, with an increase of 35% per treatment; if one day's treatment is missed, exposure should be the same as the last treatment).			
6. Complete the treatment			
a. When the treatment time is over, move the lamp away from the patient, and turn the output control to zero; dry the area with a towel.			
b. Remove material used for draping, assist the patient in dressing as needed.			
c. Clean the treatment area and equipment according to normal protocol.			

Checklist continues

PROCEDURE	Evaluation #		
	1	2	3
7. Assess treatment efficacy			
a. Ask the patient how the treated area feels.			
b. Visually inspect the treated area for any adverse reactions.			
c. Perform functional tests as indicated.			

Case Study #1: ULTRAVIOLET THERAPY

Background: A twenty-five year old man developed a psoriatic plaque over the region of the posterior aspect of his left elbow. After an unsuccessful regimen of oral medications and topical ointments his dermatologist referred him for a regimen of ultraviolet therapy. The lesion measured 3 X 5 centimeters extending over the olecranon region. The patient was otherwise in a normal state of health and exhibited full active ROM and strength of the left upper extremity.

Impression: Active psoriasis

Treatment Plan: After establishing the patient's MED (minimal erythemal dosage) as 30 seconds during an initial treatment session; a progressive program of exposure was begun to the posterior left elbow. Exposure began at 1 MED and increased by 1/2 MED each treatment session conducted on alternate days. When patient reached 6 MED exposure, treatment was suspended pending physician reassessment.

Response: There was an increase in erythema noted around the margins of the lesion subsequent to initial UV exposure. Subsequent sessions did not produce any notable change from this initial response. A gradual reduction in plaque size was noted over the course of exposures, having decreased by 30% at the time that treatment was suspended.

Case Study #2: ULTRAVIOLET THERAPY

Background: A seventy-five year old woman developed a pressure sore over the lateral malleolus of her right ankle. After an unsuccessful regimen of antibiotic medications and occlusive dressings her physician referred her for a regimen of ultraviolet therapy. The lesion measures 2 X 2 centimeters extending over the distal fibula. The patient was otherwise in a normal state of health and exhibited full active ROM and strength of the right foot and ankle.

Impression: Pressure sore

Treatment Plan: After establishing the patient's MED (minimal erythemal dosage) as 15 seconds during an initial treatment session; a progressive program of exposure was begun to the pressure sore. Exposure began at 1 MED and increased by 1/2 MED each treatment session conducted on alternate days. When the patient reached a 6 MED exposure time, treatment was suspended pending physician reassessment.

Response: There was an increase in erythema noted around the margins of the pressure sore subsequent to initial UV exposure. Subsequent exposures did not produce any notable change from this initial response. A gradual reduction in sore size was noted over the course of exposures, with the wound appearing to heal by secondary intention. Mapping of the pressure sore margin indicated a decrease of 20% in surface area at the time that treatment was suspended. Patient was subsequently referred for continuation of UV treatment until time of wound closure.

Discussion Questions for Case Studies

- What tissues were injured/affected?
- What symptoms were present?
- What phase of the injury-healing continuum did the patient present for care in?
- What are the physical agent modality's biophysical effects? (direct/indirect/depth/tissue affinity)
- What are the physical agent modality's indications/contraindications?
- What are the parameters of the physical agent modality's application/dosage/duration/frequency in this case study?

The rehabilitation professional employs physical agent modalities to create an optimum environment for tissue healing while minimizing the symptoms associated with the trauma or condition.

What other physical agent modalities could be utilized to treat this injury or condition? Why? How?

Further Discussion Questions

- Are there any medications which might sensitize the patient's response to UV?

- Are there any medical conditions which might contraindicate the use of UV for this patient's pressure sore?

- What should you do regarding treatment duration if your patient misses a scheduled treatment?

Chapter 8: LOW-POWER LASER

DESCRIPTION:

Low-power lasers produce a coherent, monochromatic, collimated light beam. They are used in the United States principally for pain modulation and wound healing. The two principal wavelengths used are 632.8 nm, produced by the helium neon (HeNe) laser, and 94 nm, produced by the gallium arsenide (GaAs) laser. Low-power (cold) lasers are distinguished from high-power (hot) lasers by the lack of thermal effects by the low-power lasers.

The mechanism of action of laser energy is not clear. Whether the absorbed photons stimulating protein synthesis, thus promoting tissue healing, have a bactericidal effect on the wound or increased angiogenesis has not been established. The potential mechanisms for pain modulation are even less clear.

Although it has been suggested that laser energy may have indirect effects on tissue up to 5 cm deep, there is no convincing evidence of penetration this deep. How light energy absorbed by the superficial cells is conducted to underlying cells when the energy is nonionizing and nonthermal has not been explained.

It should be emphasized that at this time the use of low-power lasers for these purposes has not been approved by the U.S. Food and Drug Administration, the regulating body for medical devices. Individuals using low-power lasers for these purposes must have an Investigational Device Exemption and should obtain informed consent from each patient before using the laser.

The physiologic and therapeutic effects of low-power laser stimulation are not well established. Therefore, the indications, which are derived from the physiologic effects, are somewhat speculative.

PHYSIOLOGIC EFFECTS:

- Increased collagen synthesis by fibroblasts
- Decreased nerve conduction velocity

THERAPEUTIC EFFECTS:

- Increased rate of wound closure
- Increased tensile strength of wounds
- Decreased perception of pain

INDICATIONS:

Low-power laser stimulation may be helpful to optimize the rate of wound closure, modulate musculoskeletal pain, and remodel established scar tissue.

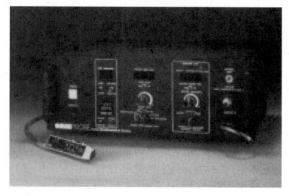 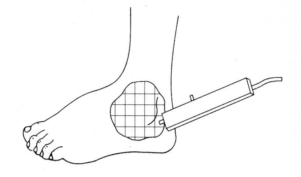

PhysioTechnology, Ltd. Topeka, Kans.

CONTRAINDICATIONS:

There are no established contraindications to low-power laser application, but the light should not be directed at the eyes.

LOW-POWER LASER

PROCEDURE	Evaluation #		
	1	2	3
1. Check supplies			
a. Obtain sheet or towels for draping, protective goggles for patient and therapist as required.			
b. Check laser equipment for charged battery, broken or frayed cables, and integrity of shields.			
2. Question patient			
a. Verify identity of patient (if not already verified).			
b. Verify the absence of contraindications.			
c. Ask about previous exposure to laser therapy, check treatment notes.			
3. Position patient			
a. Place patient in a well-supported, comfortable position.			

Checklist continues

PROCEDURE	Evaluation #		
	1	2	3
b. Expose body part to be treated.			
c. Drape patient to preserve patient's modesty, protect clothing, but allow access to body part.			
4. Inspect body part to be treated			
a. Check light touch perception.			
b. Assess function of body part (e.g., ROM, irritability).			
5. Apply laser stimulation.			
a. Determine the area to be treated and visualize a grid overlying the treatment area. The grid should be divided into 1-cm squares.			
b. If the gridding technique is to be used, place the tip of the probe in light contact with the skin and administer the light to each square centimeter of area for the appropriate time to obtain the desired dosage.			
c. If the scanning technique is to be used, hold the tip of the probe within 1 cm of the skin and make sure the aperture of the probe is positioned such that the laser beam will be perpendicular to the skin. Administer the light to each square centimeter of area for the appropriate time to obtain the desired dosage.			
d. Insure that the laser energy will not be directed at the patient's eyes.			
e. If the patient reports anything unusual, such as discomfort at the treatment site, nausea or dizzines; discontinue treatment.			

Checklist continues

PROCEDURE	Evaluation #		
	1	2	3
f. Continue to monitor the patient for the duration of the treatment.			
6. Complete the treatment			
a. When the treatment time is over, discontinue application of the laser energy.			
b. Remove material used for draping, assist the patient in dressing as needed.			
c. Have the patient perform appropriate therapeutic exercise as indicated.			
d. Clean the treatment area and equipment according to normal protocol.			
7. Assess treatment efficacy.			
a. Ask the patient how the treated area feels.			
b. Visually inspect the treated area for any adverse reactions.			
c. Perform functional tests as indicated.			

Case Study: LOW-POWER LASER

Background: A 44 year-old man who has had Type I diabetes mellitus for 30 years presents for treatment of a non- or slow-healing lesion on his left foot. He has a mild peripheral sensory neuropathy, and developed a blister after going for a long run with new running shoes. The initial injury occurred 3 months ago, and there has been no change in the size of the lesion for the past month. The lesion is on the plantar surface of the foot, under the first metatarsal head. It is a full-thickness lesion, and is approximately 3 cm in diameter. The patient's medical condition is stable, and there are no other complaints.

Impression: Chronic dermal lesion on the left foot.

Treatment Plan: Daily treatment with a Helium-Neon laser was initiated. After cleansing the wound under aseptic conditions, the entire lesion was exposed to the HeNe light at 632.8 nm wavelength. The scanning technique was used to prevent contamination of the wound and equipment. The entire lesion was treated with an energy density of 4.0 Joules per square centimeter.

Response: Photographs were taken on a weekly basis to document the effects of the treatment. After 3 weeks of daily treatment, the frequency was decreased to 3 sessions per week. After a total of 21 sessions (5 weeks), the lesion was healed. The patient was taught self-care, and techniques to prevent further injuries.

Discussion Questions for Case Study

- What tissues were injured/affected?
- What symptoms were present?
- What phase of the injury-healing continuum did the patient present for care in?
- What are the physical agent modality's biophysical effects? (direct/indirect/depth/tissue affinity)
- What are the physical agent modality's indications/contraindications?
- What are the parameters of the physical agent modality's application/dosage/duration/frequency in this case study?

    The rehabilitation professional employs physical agent modalities to create an optimum environment for tissue healing while minimizing the symptoms associated with the trauma or condition.
    What other physical agent modalities could be utilized to treat this injury or condition? Why? How?

Further Discussion Questions

- What is the mechanism of action of the laser energy?

- Why are patients with diabetes mellitus susceptible to cutaneous lesions?

- What precautions must be taken before treating a patient with a low-powered laser?

- What alternative treatment techniques would you consider?

- What are their advantages and disadvantages as compared to using a laser?

Chapter 9: THERAPEUTIC ULTRASOUND

DESCRIPTION:

Therapeutic ultrasound is a physical agent modality most frequently utilized in sports medicine for the purpose of elevating tissue temperature, stimulating the repair of musculoskeletal soft tissues, modulating pain and in the case of phonophoresis, driving medicinal molecules into a local tissue. Ultrasound is a high frequency, inaudible acoustic sound wave that may produce either thermal or non-thermal physiologic effects within the body. When applied to biologic tissues ultrasound may induce significant responses in cells, tissues and organs. Ultrasound is one of the most widely utilized physical agent modalities in addition to the thermotherapies and electrotherapies.

PHYSIOLOGICAL EFFECTS:

- Thermal effects
    - Elevated tissue temperature
    - Increased blood flow
    - Increased tissue extensibility
    - Increased local metabolism
    - Altered nerve conduction velocity
- Non-thermal effects
    - Cavitation
        - Fluid movement
            - Increased cellular membrane permeability
    - Acoustic microstreaming
        - Stimulation of fibroblast activity

THERAPEUTIC EFFECTS:

- Increased collagen tissues extensibility
- Decreased joint stiffness
- Reduction of muscle spasm
- Modulation of pain
- Increased blood flow
- Mild inflammatory response
- Stimulation of tissue regeneration

INDICATIONS:

The primary indication for the use of therapeutic ultrasound by the sports therapist is in the acute and chronic treatment of soft tissue dysfunction, i.e., strains, sprains, contusions with associated symptoms of pain and muscular spasm. Ultrasound has also been successfully employed to enhance soft tissue and bone healing. Ultrasound can also be employed to percutaneously deliver selected medications to areas of inflammation.

CONTRAINDICATIONS:

- Areas of impaired pain or temperature sensation
- Areas of impaired circulation
- Epiphyseal areas in children
- Not over reproductive organs
- Not over eyes, heart, spinal cord or cervical/stellate ganglia
- Not over cemented joint prostheses
- Not over malignancies

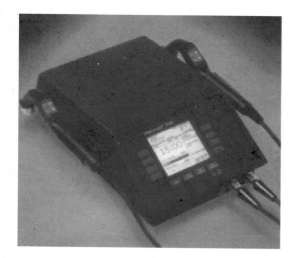

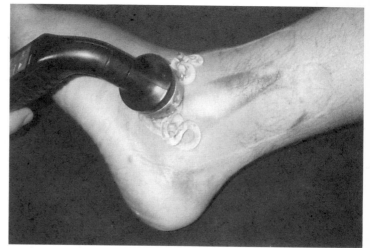

Manufactured by Physio Technology Inc., Topeka, Kans.

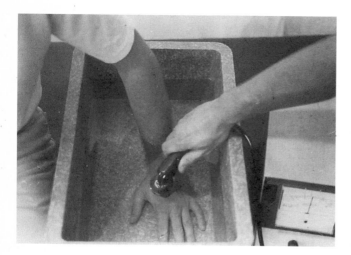

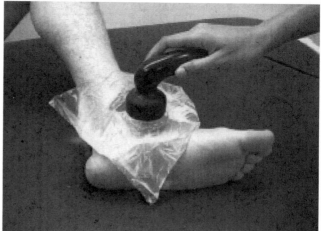

THERAPE UTIC ULTRASOUND

PROCEDURE	Evaluation #		
	1	2	3
1. Check supplies and equipment			
a. Obtain appropriate ultrasound unit (1 or 3 Mhz), towels, and coupling gel			
2. Question patient			
a. Verify identity of patient			
b. Verify the absence of contraindications			
c. Ask about previous ultrasound treatments and check previous treatment notes			
3. Position patient			
a. Place patient in a well-supported, comfortable position			
b. Expose body part to be treated			
c. Drape patient to preserve patient's modesty, protect clothing, but allow access to body part			
4. Inspect body part to be treated			
a. Check sensation			
b. Check circulatory status			
c. Verify that there are no rashes or open wounds			
d. Assess function of body part (e.g., ROM, strength, irritability)			
5. Apply indicated technique: Select Continuous or Pulsed Output and verify output intensity is at 0 before turning unit power on			

Checklist continues

a. Direct Coupling			
1. Apply layer of coupling gel to treatment surface			
2. Establish treatment duration dependent upon size of area to be treated (i.e., 5 minutes for each 16 square inch area)			
3. Maintain contact between sound head and treatment surface, moving sound head in circular or linear overlapping strokes at a rate of 2 - 4 inches per second - observe for air bubble formation			
4. Adjust treatment intensity: .5 - 1.0 watts/cm^2 for superficial tissues and 1.0 - 2.0 watts/cm^2 for deeper tissues			
5. Monitor patient response during treatment - if patient reports warmth or ache - reduce intensity by 10% and continue treatment			
b. Bladder Coupling			
1. Fill a balloon or condom with tepid, degassed water			
2. Apply layer of coupling gel to bladder			
3. Apply layer of coupling gel to treatment surface			
4. Place bladder over treatment surface			
5. Establish treatment duration dependent upon size of area to be treated (i.e., 5 minutes for each 16 square inch area)			

Checklist continues

6.	Maintain contact between sound head and treatment surface, moving sound head in circular or linear overlapping strokes at a rate of 2 - 4 inches per second - observe for air bubble formation			
7.	Adjust treatment intensity: .5 - 1.0 watts/cm^2 for superficial tissues and 1.0 - 2.0 watts/cm^2 for deeper tissues, intensity may need to be increased			
8.	Monitor patient response during treatment - if patient reports warmth or ache - reduce intensity by 10% and continue treatment			
c. **Underwater Coupling**				
1.	Fill a plastic or ceramic non-conductive basin with tepid degassed water of sufficient depth to cover treatment surface			
2.	Immerse the body part into the basin			
3.	Establish treatment duration dependent upon size of area to be treated (i.e., 5 minutes for each 16 square inch area)			
4.	Maintain sound head parallel to treatment surface at a distance of .5 - 3 cm, moving sound head in circular or linear overlapping strokes at a rate of 2 - 4 inches per second - observe for air bubble formation on sound head and wipe away			

Checklist continues

5.	Adjust treatment intensity: .5 - 1.0 watts/cm^2 for superficial tissues and 1.0 - 2.0 watts/cm^2 for deeper tissues, intensity may need to be increased			
6.	Monitor patient response during treatment - if patient reports warmth or ache - reduce intensity by 10% and continue treatment			
d. **Phonophoresis**				
1.	Cleanse treatment surface with alcohol or soap and water			
2.	Apply medication in glycerol cream, oil or other vehicle in lieu of coupling gel			
3.	Establish treatment duration dependent upon size of area to be treated (i.e., 5 minutes for each 16 square inch area)			
4.	Maintain contact between sound head and treatment surface, moving sound head in circular or linear overlapping strokes at a rate of 2 - 4 inches per second - observe for air bubble formation			
5.	Adjust treatment intensity: .5 - 1.0 watts/cm^2 for superficial tissues and 1.0 - 2.0 watts/cm^2 for deeper tissues, intensity may need to be decreased			

Checklist continues

	6.	Monitor patient response during treatment - if patient reports warmth or ache - reduce intensity by 10% continue treatment			
6.	Terminate treatment				
	a.	Zero out ultrasound unit control before removing sound head			
	b.	Clean sound head of excess gel or medication in vehicle			
	c.	Clean treatment surface of excess gel or medication in vehicle			
	d.	Visually inspect the treated area			
	e.	Remove draping material and have patient dress			
7.	Assess treatment efficacy				
	a.	Ask the patient how treated area feels			
	b.	Record treatment parameters			
8.	Instruct the patient in any indicated exercise				
9.	Return equipment to storage after cleaning				

Case Study #1: THERAPEUTIC ULTRASOUND

Background: An eighteen year old college freshman sustained a fracture of the fifth metacarpal of the left hand during a prank in the dormitory. The fracture required gauntlet cast immobilization for six weeks. At the time of cast removal the patient noted significant restriction of motion and weakness in the left wrist. A referral was initiated. Physical examination revealed flexion 0 to 45 degrees, extension 0 to 30 degrees with radial and ulnar deviation unaffected. There was point tenderness at the callus site on the shaft of the fifth metacarpal. Finger motion was grossly within normal limits at all constituent joints.

Impression: Wrist capsule motion restriction secondary to immobilization, muscular weakness secondary to immobilization.

Treatment Plan: A course of therapeutic ultrasound was initiated to decrease joint stiffness through increased collagen-connective tissue extensibility. Given the small and irregular surface of the wrist joint, underwater coupling was chosen as the mode of ultrasound delivery. After checking the left wrist and hand for any rashes or open wounds and verifying that sensation and circulation were normal in the distal portion of the extremity; the left forearm, wrist and hand were immersed in a plastic basin filled with warm water. An ultrasound treatment of 1.5 watts/cm^2 for 6 minutes was applied to the dorsal aspect of the left wrist. Patient reported a mild sensation of warmth. At the conclusion of the treatment the patient was instructed in active and active-assistive wrist mobilization exercises.

Response: Following initial US treatment and exercise patient experienced a 10 degree improvement in both flexion and extension range of motion. At the completion of the sixth treatment wrist range of motion was within normal limits and the patient was aggressively pursuing a wrist curl strengthening regimen. Ultrasound treatments were discontinued at that time with efforts focused on strengthening and functional use of the left upper extremity.

Case Study #2: THERAPEUTIC ULTRASOUND

Background: A twelve year old junior high school student sustained a deep bruise of the left quadriceps muscle in a fall from his skateboard. The parents were advised by their pediatrician to apply cold initially and then moist heat until the problem resolved. At this time, some one month post-injury there remains significant restriction of left knee motion. A referral was initiated to physical therapy at the parent's request. Physical examination revealed active knee motion of only 10 to 65 degrees. There was point tenderness and a well demarcated hematoma palpable in the middle third of the vastus lateralis.

Impression: Knee motion restriction secondary to soft tissue contusion and hematoma formation.

Treatment Plan: A course of pulsed therapeutic ultrasound was initiated to decrease the hematoma formation through increased collagen-connective tissue extensibility and reabsorption of the extracellular debrise from the original contusion. Patient reported a mild sensation of warmth. At the conclusion of the treatment the patient was instructed in active and active-assistive knee range of motion exercises.

Response: Following initial US treatment and exercise patient experienced a 10 degree improvement in knee flexion and extension range of motion. At the completion of the tenth treatment session knee range of motion was within normal limits and the patient was aggressively pursuing a quadriceps strengthening regimen. Ultrasound treatments were discontinued at that time with efforts focused on strengthening and functional use of the left lower extremity.

Discussion Questions for Case Studies

- What tissues were injured/affected?
- What symptoms were present?
- What phase of the injury-healing continuum did the patient present for care in?
- What are the physical agent modality's biophysical effects? (direct/indirect/depth/tissue affinity)
- What are the physical agent modality's indications/contraindications?
- What are the parameters of the physical agent modality's application/dosage/duration/frequency in this case study?

The rehabilitation professional employs physical agent modalities to create an optimum environment for tissue healing while minimizing the symptoms associated with the trauma or condition.

What other physical agent modalities could be utilized to treat this injury or condition? Why? How?

Further Discussion Questions

- Which ultrasound frequency would be optimal for this patient's condition?

- What would be your response to the patient's complaint of a dull ache during the treatment?

- Because of the patients' ages are there any additional precautions you should take in utilizing ultrasound?

Chapter 10: MECHANICAL TRACTION

DESCRIPTION: Mechanical traction has been used since ancient times in the treatment of painful spinal conditions. Simply traction is applying tension to a body segment though a rope attached to various straps, halters or devices. The therapeutic effect of traction is a function of the position of the spine, amount of traction force and length of time the force is applied. Mechanical traction results in longitudinal separation of cervical or lumbar spinal segments with associated ligament, diskal, neural and muscular structures.

THERAPEUTIC EFFECTS:

- Separation of Spinal Segments
- Elongation of Muscle, Ligament and Capsular Tissue
- Reduced Intradiscal Pressure

INDICATIONS:

Mechanical traction is indicated to reduce the signs and symptoms of spinal compression. Appropriately applied mechanical traction can stretch facet joint capsules, increase the dimension of the intervertebral foramen thus increasing space for nerve roots, and alter intradiscal pressure. Paraspinal muscle tissues can also be elongated contributing to a reduction in the pain/spasm cycle which frequently accompanies spinal dysfunction.

CONTRAINDICATIONS:

- Spinal infection or malignancy
- Rheumatoid arthritis
- Osteoporosis
- Spinal hypermobility
- Acute stage injury
- Cardiac or respiratory insufficiency
- Pregnancy

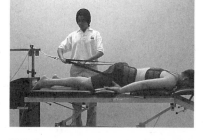

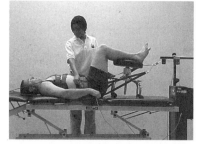

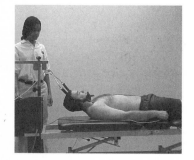

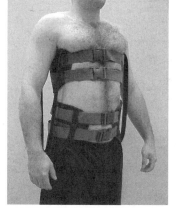

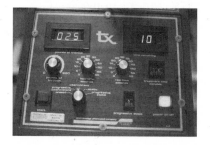

MECHANICAL TRACTION

PROCEDURE	Evaluation #		
	1	2	3
1. Check supplies and equipment			
a. Assemble towels, halters, harnesses and belts			
2. Question patient			
a. Verify identity of patient			
b. Verify the absence of contraindications			
c. Ask about previous traction treatments and review treatment record			
3. Apply and adjust appropriate halters, harnesses and belts for indicated traction treatment			
a. Cervical - apply head halter beneath the occiput and mandible, attach to spreader bar			
b. Lumbar - attach pelvic harness snugly about the waist beginning just above the iliac crests, thoracic rib belt snugly about the lower rib cage			
c. Attach traction apparatus to unit - take up and adjust for slack in the line			
4. Position patient for indicated traction treatment			
a. Cervical - supine lying with neck flexed 20 - 30 degrees			
b. Lumbar - supine hooklying with hips flexed and legs supported by pillows or stools			
c. Lumbar - prone lying in neutral			
d. Insure proper body alignment and pull of traction apparatus			

Checklist continues

4.		Apply indicated traction poundage			
	a.	Cervical - adjust traction poundage beginning with 20# or as tolerated by the patient, (range 20 -> 50 pounds)			
	b.	Lumbar - adjust traction poundage beginning with 65# or as tolerated by the patient (range 65 -> 200 pounds)			
5.		Adjust traction duty cycle and treatment duration			
	a.	Sustained - $\leq$ 10 minutes			
	b.	Intermittent - 3 to 10 seconds on/off for 20 -> 30 minutes			
6.		Complete the Treatment			
	a.	Zero out equipment, turn power off			
	b.	Slacken traction line			
	c.	Remove the traction harness, halter or belt			
	d.	Have patient sit up slowly			
	e.	Assess treatment efficacy			
	f.	Record treatment parameters			
7.		Instruct the patient in any indicated exercise			
8.		Return equipment to storage after cleaning			

Case Study: MECHANICAL TRACTION

Background: A 49 year-old man developed lower cervical pain 4 days ago following a pick-up game of basketball; although the patient runs on a regular basis, playing basketball is not part of his normal exercise regimen. He has been referred for symptomatic treatment of his mechanical neck pain; there are no neural deficits, and no signs of a disk lesion. The patient is experiencing pain in the midline of the lower cervical area, and across the upper trapezius area bilaterally. His active range of motion is normal, but is painful at the end of range in all planes, and overpressure increases the symptoms. Extension (back bending) is the most painful motion.

Impression: Soft-tissue injury of the lower cervical spine.

Treatment Plan: To assist in pain relief, a 3-day per week course of intermittent mechanical cervical traction was initiated. The patient was positioned supine on the traction table, and the traction unit was adjusted to produce approximately 20 degrees of cervical flexion during traction. For the initial session, 20 pounds of traction was applied, with 4 progressive steps up, and 4 regressive steps down. Each traction cycle consisted of 15 seconds of tension, followed by 20 seconds of rest. Total treatment time was 20 minutes. The target traction force was increased by 10% each session, to a maximum of 40 pounds. In addition to the traction, active exercise was prescribed.

Response: The patient reported a transient increase in symptoms following the first two sessions, then a gradual resolution of the symptoms. There was a marked reduction in symptoms immediately following the third session; the relief persisted for approximately 2 hours. Cervical traction was discontinued after a total of 6 sessions, and the patient was instructed in a home exercise program. Two weeks later, the patient was asymptomatic.

Discussion Questions for Case Study

- What tissues were injured/affected?
- What symptoms were present?
- What phase of the injury-healing continuum did the patient present for care in?
- What are the physical agent modality's biophysical effects? (direct/indirect/depth/tissue affinity)
- What are the physical agent modality's indications/contraindications?
- What are the parameters of the physical agent modality's application/dosage/duration/frequency in this case study?

The rehabilitation professional employs physical agent modalities to create an optimum environment for tissue healing while minimizing the symptoms associated with the trauma or condition.

What other physical agent modalities could be utilized to treat this injury or condition? Why? How?

Further Discussion Questions

- What was the mechanism of injury to the cervical spine?

- What were the physiological effects of the cervical traction?

- Why was the supine position used for the treatment?

- What additional physical agents may have been helpful for this patient?

- What are the contraindications to cervical traction?

- Why were the patient's symptoms initially increased?

Chapter 11: INTERMITTENT COMPRESSION

DESCRIPTION:

Intermittent compression pumps are mechanical units which inflate double-layered fabric sleeves shaped to fit the extremities in order to apply external pressure to facilitate the body's reabsorption of edema resulting from injury or trauma. Units allow the regulation of inflation pressure, on/off time sequence and total treatment time.

PHYSIOLOGICAL EFFECTS:

- Movement of interstitial fluid to venous and lymphatic drainage sites
- Temporary decrease in peripheral blood flow

THERAPEUTIC EFFECTS:

- Reduction of soft tissue edema
- Decreased pain
- Increased range of motion

INDICATIONS:

The sports therapist will most frequently employ intermittent compression pumps in the treatment of soft tissue edema or intra-articular effusion which accompanies musculoskeletal trauma. It may also be utilized in cases of venous insufficiency and lymphedema.

CONTRAINDICATIONS:

- Infections
- Arterial Insufficiency
- Possibility of blood clots
- Cardiac or kidney dysfunction
- Obstructed lymphatic channels

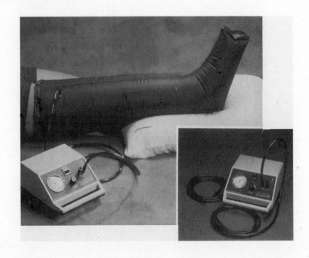

INTERMITTENT COMPRESSION

PROCEDURE	Evaluation #		
	1	2	3
1. Check Supplies			
a. Obtain compression pump, pneumatic sleeve, and cotton stockingnette			
2. Question Patient			
a. Verify identity of patient			
b. Verify the absence of contraindications			
c. Take the patient's blood pressure			
d. Ask about previous treatments and review treatment notes			
3. Position Patient			
a. Place patient in a well-supported, comfortable position			
b. Elevate the extremity to be treated			
4. Inspect the patient's skin and extremity sensation			
a. Perform circumferential measures of part to be treated			
b. Cover extremity with stockingnette, insure there are no wrinkles			
5. Apply compression sleeve over the stockingnette-covered extremity			
6. Explain the procedure to patient			

Checklist continues

7.	Begin the indicated procedure			
	a.	Attach sleeve to compression pump via tubing			
	b.	Turn pump "on" and inflate to: $\leq$ 60mm for the lower extremity $\leq$ 50mm for the upper extremity DO NOT EXCEED DIASTOLIC BP			
	c.	Adjust the compression pump to cycle in a 3:1 ratio of on and off time			
	d.	Set duration of treatment from 30 minutes to one hour			
	e.	Encourage the patient to wiggle their fingers or toes during the off cycle			
	f.	Remove the sleeve at least once during the course of treatment to inspect skin and allow joint motion			
8.	Complete the Treatment			
	a.	Remove the sleeve and stockingnette			
	b.	Inspect the skin and check peripheral circulation			
	c.	Perform circumferential measures			
	d.	Record results of treatment			
	e.	Assess treatment efficacy			
9.	Wrap extremity to retain edema reduction and perform any indicated exercise			
10.	Return equipment to storage after cleaning			

Case Study #1: INTERMITTENT COMPRESSION

Background: A 48-year-old male developed pain and edema in his right foot and ankle subsequent to stepping in a hole in his yard while mowing his lawn. Treated at his local hospital's emergency room; he failed to comply with their instructions to elevate and ice the injured extremity and reported to his family physician 48 hours later with a moderately swollen and ecchymotic right ankle. The patient reported the obvious swelling, localized tenderness over the lateral aspect of the ankle and difficulty with weight-bearing during ambulation. Physical examination revealed point tenderness at the ATF (anterior talofibular ligament), 2+ effusion - figure 8 girth increased by 3/4" versus uninvolved side, and reduced ROM of dorsiflexion to 0 degrees/plantarflexion to 35 degrees. The ankle was stable to anterior drawer and talar tilt tests.

Impression: Subacute grade I inversion sprain right ankle

Treatment Plan: In addition to reinstruction in home care principles; a course of intermittent compression was initiated to the right foot/ankle to mobilize the residual effusion/edema. The right lower extremity was elevated, pre-treatment circumferential measurements taken and stockingnette placed over the extremity. Treatment consisted of 60mm Hg pressure applied intermittently for 30 seconds on/10 seconds off cycles for 30 minutes duration. Post-treatment circumferential measures were taken and the patient encouraged to attempt active and active-assisted ankle pumping exercise. Patient was fitted with a compression stocking and thermoplastic ankle stirrup for ambulation weight-bearing as tolerated.

Response: Post initial treatment, patient's circumferential measures were reduced by 1/4". Dorsiflexion range of motion increased by 5 degrees. Over the course of five treatment sessions, effusion was resolved and active range of motion approached normal limits. Strengthening exercises were implemented and the patient continued to ambulate with the aid of the ankle stirrup. At the time of discharge the patient was essentially symptom free, independent in performing his strengthening regimen and had returned to his yard work.

Case Study #2: INTERMITTENT COMPRESSION

Background: A 32-year-old woman underwent a modified radical mastectomy on the right 1 year ago, followed by radiation treatment for breast cancer. She had done well until approximately 6 months ago, when she began participation in a breast cancer survivor rowing team. Since then, she developed swelling in the right upper member, from the hand to the axilla. The swelling is beginning to interfere with her normal daily activities and the rowing. She has been referred for assistance in management of the edema. Circumferential measurements of her upper members reveals that the right upper member is 20 percent larger than the left upper member; this difference is constant from the deltoid tubercle to the wrist.

Impression: Postmastecomy lymphedema syndrome due to lymph node removal and radiation damage.

Treatment Plan: Intermittent compression using a full-length upper extremity sleeve. The inflation pressure was initially set at 40 mmHg, with an on time of 45 seconds, and off time of 60 seconds, and a total treatment time of 30 minutes. The patient was positioned supine, with the right upper member elevated on pillows, and she was asked to make and release a fist during the time the sleeve was deflated. Treatment was conducted 3 days per week for a total of 15 sessions.

Response: There was a slight decrease in right upper member circumference following the initial treatment, but the reduction was not maintained. Over the next three sessions, the maximum inflation pressure was gradually increased to 60 mmHg, and the on time was increased to 120 seconds, with an off time of 30 seconds. There was a steady decrease in limb circumference until the 11th session, after which there were no further gains noted. She was then fitted with a custom elastic garment to assist in maintaining the reduced limb volume. Upon discharge, her right upper member had a circumference that was 8 percent greater than the left upper member.

Discussion Questions for Case Studies

- What tissues were injured/affected?
- What symptoms were present?
- What phase of the injury-healing continuum did the patient present for care in?
- What are the physical agent modality's biophysical effects? (direct/indirect/depth/tissue affinity)
- What are the physical agent modality's indications/contraindications?
- What are the parameters of the physical agent modality's application/dosage/duration/frequency in this case study?

The rehabilitation professional employs physical agent modalities to create an optimum environment for tissue healing while minimizing the symptoms associated with the trauma or condition.

What other physical agent modalities could be utilized to treat this injury or condition? Why? How?

Further Discussion Questions

- How would you maintain the reduction in foot/ankle swelling obtained from the intermittent compression?

- If the patient reported tingling or numbness in his toes during treatment what would be your response?

- What is the difference in the pathophysiology of postmastectomy lymphedema and the edema noted with musculoskeletal injuries? If there a difference in treatment techniques? Duration of treatment? Probability of recurrence?

- Would this patient have been more or less likely to develop lymphedema if she had undergone a simple mastectomy? A radical mastectomy?

- What effect did the radiation therapy have on the development of lymphedema? Would a course of chemotherapy have had the same effect? Why or why not?

- Could the development of postmastectomy lymphedema have been prevented in this patient? Why or why not? What measures could have been used in a attempt to prevent the lymphedema?

- What was the rationale for having the limb elevated during the intermittent compression? For the making and releasing a fist? For intermittent as opposed to static compression? For the inflation pressure?

- Would an inflation pressure of 120 mmHg have been more effective at reducing the edema?

Chapter 12: MASSAGE

DESCRIPTION:

Massage is most likely the oldest form of mechanical therapy for injury. Even very small children know that rubbing an injured area tends to diminish the pain. As with essentially all physical agents, the massage itself does not produce healing, but the therapeutic effects can assist during the healing process.

There are many types of massage, each with proponents and detractors. The different types of massage have different proposed physiological and therapeutic effects, though there is a great deal of overlap. In essence, all forms of massage involve the application of mechanical force to various tissues of the body, usually with the therapist's hands. Massage may exert an influence on the injured or dysfunctional tissue either via a direct mechanical action or via neurological reflexes.

PHYSIOLOGICAL EFFECTS:

- Increase in large diameter afferent neural input
- Increase in venous outflow
- Increase in lymph outflow

THERAPEUTIC EFFECTS:

- Decreased pain
- Decreased soft tissue swelling and congestion
- Remodeling of collagen

INDICATIONS:

The indications for massage vary depending on the type of massage used. In general, pain, swelling, and connective tissue contracture are the indications for massage.

CONTRAINDICATIONS:

There are no absolute contraindications to massage. Obviously, precautions should be used in the case of fractures, open wounds, and severe pain. The amount of pressure applied can be regulated based upon the irritability of the tissue and the desired therapeutic effect sought.

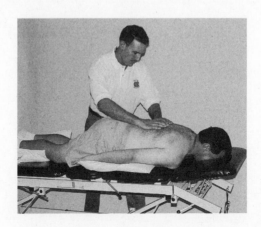

MASSAGE

PROCEDURE	Evaluation #		
	1	2	3
1. Check supplies			
a. Obtain sheet or towels for draping.			
b. Obtain lubricant as indicated			
2. Question patient			
a. Verify identity of patient (if not already verified).			
b. Verify the absence of contraindications.			
c. Ask about previous massage treatments, check treatment notes.			
3. Position patient			
a. Place patient in a well-supported, comfortable position. Positioning is particularly crucial for massage.			
b. Expose body part to be treated.			
c. Drape patient to preserve patient's modesty, protect clothing, but allow access to body part.			
4. Inspect body part to be treated			
a. Check light touch perception.			
b. Check circulatory status (pulses, capillary refill).			
c. Verify that there are no open wounds or rashes.			
d. Assess function of body part (e.g., ROM, irritability).			

Checklist continues

PROCEDURE	Evaluation #		
	1	2	3
5a. Apply Hoffa massage			
a. After applying lubricant, **effleurage** is applied with a stroking motion from distal to proximal with light to moderate pressure; the deeper tissue is not moved. The initial strokes serve to distribute the lubricant over the treatment area.			
b. **Petrissage** is a kneading type motion, where the muscles are lifted and rolled.			
c. **Tapotement** is a series of percussion movements with the tips of the fingers, the ulnar border of the hands, the heel of the hands, or cupped hands.			
d. **Vibration** is a rapid oscillation or tremor of the hands when they are in firm contact with the skin.			
5b. Apply **transverse friction** massage			
a. No lubricant is used.			
b. The tendon or ligament is placed on a slight stretch.			
c. Using deep pressure such that the skin and thumb or finger move together over the deeper tissue, apply a back-and-forth motion perpendicular to the fibers of the tendon or ligament.			
d. The duration of the massage should be up to 10 minutes, or as tolerated by the patient.			

Checklist continues

PROCEDURE	Evaluation #		
	1	2	3
5c. Apply connective tissue massage (**Bindegewebsmassage**)			
a. No lubricant is used			
b. Using the tips of the third and fourth digits, the skin and subcutaneous tissues are pulled away from the fascia.			
c. The massage extends from the coccyx to the upper lumbar area, and each pulling stroke should produce a transient, sharp pain.			
d. Duration of treatment should be 15 to 25 minutes or as tolerated by the patient.			
5d. Acupressure/Trigger Point Massage			
a. No lubricant is used.			
b. Technique is similar to transverse friction massage, but is applied to a trigger or acupuncture point (found using a chart, or by palpation). Trigger points usually are nodular-like lumps in a muscle, and often feel gritty.			
c. Using the tip of any digit, or even the olecranon process, the skin is moved on the trigger point; no motion should take place between the therapist and the patient's skin. The motion is circular, and is confined to the point.			
d. Pressure will be painful, and as hard as the patient can tolerate. The pressure may produce pain radiating to distant areas.			
e. Duration of the massage is between one and five minutes per point.			

Checklist continues

PROCEDURE	Evaluation #		
	1	2	3
6. Complete treatment			
a. Upon completion of the massage, remove any lubricant with a towel.			
b. Remove material used for draping, assist the patient in dressing as needed.			
c. Have the patient perform appropriate therapeutic exercise indicated.			
d. Clean the treatment area and equipment according to normal protocol.			
7. Assess treatment efficacy			
a. Ask the patient how the treated area feels.			
b. Visually inspect the treated area for any adverse reactions.			
c. Perform functional tests as indicated.			

Case Study: MASSAGE

Background: A thirty-year old stockbroker complains of chronic cervical myalgia ("my neck hurts"). There was no prior history of trauma and his family physician reported that his radiographs were within normal limits without evidence of degenerative changes or loss of disk space height. The patient reported no radiation of pain into the shoulders or upper extremities, but did complain of restriction in rotating his head to the left. The patient states that he spends many hours each day at work cradling a telephone with his right side.

Impression: "Occupational Neck" - Right Upper Trapezius and Sternocleidomastoid Muscle Spasm

Treatment Plan: The patient was placed in a forward seated position with the head and neck supported by pillows on the treatment plinth. The arms were likewise supported by a pillow in the lap. A small amount of prewarmed massage lotion was applied to the right upper quarter region and a Hoffa massage commenced with light effleurage stroking begun to the SCM and upper trapezius muscles. The light effleurage stroking was followed by several minutes of deep effleurage strokes which identified several 'trigger point' areas in each muscle. Petrissage was directed at each 'trigger point' area for approximately 30 seconds then the massage concluded with several more minutes of deep then superficial effleurage strokes. At the completion of the massage, excess lotion was removed then the patient instructed in cervical and upper quarter active range of motion exercise. The patient was encouraged to perform his home range of motion exercises each AM and PM.

Response: The patient reported immediate relief of his symptoms following the initial session of massage. He reported the ability to fully turn and bend his head and neck. The patient returned for two additional sessions of massage treatment and was educated as to postural habits that triggered his condition. He continued his BID range of motion exercises, added isometric strengthening exercises to his daily regimen and monitored his postural habits at work. His employer subsequently added once weekly visits by a massage therapist as an employee benefit.

Discussion Questions for Case Study

- What tissues were injured/affected?
- What symptoms were present?
- What phase of the injury-healing continuum did the patient present for care in?
- What are the physical agent modality's biophysical effects? (direct/indirect/depth/tissue affinity)
- What are the physical agent modality's indications/contraindications?
- What are the parameters of the physical agent modality's application/dosage/duration/frequency in this case study?

The rehabilitation professional employs physical agent modalities to create an optimum environment for tissue healing while minimizing the symptoms associated with the trauma or condition.

What other physical agent modalities could be utilized to treat this injury or condition? Why? How?

Further Discussion Questions

- When would you discontinue massage?

- If the patient reported a rash subsequent to the initial massage treatment your response would be?

SELECTED REFERENCES

Belanger, AY. 2002. *Evidence based guide to therapeutic physical agents.* Philadelphia, PA: Lippincott-Williams & Wilkens,

Cameron, MH. 1999. *Physical agents in rehabilitation.* Philadelphia, PA: W.B. Saunders.

Gersh, M. 1992. Vol. 7. *Electrotherapy in rehabilitation.* Philadelphia, PA: F.A. Davis.

Griffen, JE. 1988. *Physical agents for physical therapists.* 3rd ed. La Crescenta, CA: C.C .Thomas.

Hayes, K.W. 1993. *Manual for physical agents.* 4th ed. East Norwalk, CT: Appleton & Lange.

Kahn, J. 1991. *Principles and practice of electrotherapy.* 2d ed. New York, NY: Churchill-Livingstone.

Knight, K.L. 1995. *Cryotherapy in sports injury management.* Champaign, IL: Human Kinetics.

Lehman, J.F. 1988. *Therapeutic heat and cold.* 3d ed. Baltimore, MD: Williams & Wilkins.

Michlovitz, S. 1996. *Thermal agents in rehabilitation.* 3d ed. Philadelphia, PA: F.A. Davis.

Nelson, R., and Currier, D. 1991. *Clinical electrotherapy.* 2d ed. East Norwalk, CT: Appleton & Lange.

Prentice, W. 2002. *Therapeutic modalities in sports medicine and athletic training.* 5th ed. New York, NY: McGraw-Hill.

Snyder-Mackler, L., and Robinson, A. 1995. *Clinical electrophysiology: electrotherapy and electrophysiologic testing.* 2nd ed. Baltimore, MD: Williams & Wilkins.